THE
PATIENT
PARADOX

THE
PATIENT
PARADOX

Why sexed-up medicine is
bad for your health

Margaret McCartney

The Patient Paradox
Why sexed-up medicine is bad for your health

First published in Great Britain by Pinter & Martin Ltd 2012
reprinted 2013

ISBN 978-1-78066-000-4

Also available as an ebook

British Library Cataloguing-in-Publication Data
A catalogue record for this book is available from the British Library

Printed in Great Britain by TJ International Ltd, Padstow, Cornwall

This book has been printed on paper that is sourced and harvested from
sustainable forests and is FSC accredited

Pinter & Martin Ltd
6 Effra Parade
London SW2 1PS

www.pinterandmartin.com
www.thepatientparadox.com

For Joseph, Agnes and Jude

About the author

Margaret McCartney is a GP in Glasgow, and has three children. She started writing for the press after being infuriated by an article in a newspaper which claimed that CT body screening was the way to stay well. Since then she has written for most UK newspapers, as well as the *British Medical Journal (BMJ)*, other magazines such as *Vogue* and *Prospect*, has had columns in the *Guardian* and the *FT Weekend*, and is a regular contributor to BBC Radio 4's *Inside Health*. She has won prizes from the Medical Journalists' Association and the European School of Oncology, as well as the Healthwatch award.

She has a strong interest in evidence, professionalism, screening and risk. She blogs and tweets. *The Patient Paradox* is her first book.

www.margaretmccartney.com/blog
Twitter @mgtmccartney

Acknowledgements

With very many thanks to my publisher Martin Wagner, my editor Jonathan Lalljee, and my husband Cónal, for their collective encouragement, conviction and wisdom. My parents have supported and helped me in numerous invaluable ways. The people who have inspired and educated my understanding and practice of medicine are many, and most are named, or their work is cited, in this book.

Contents

Introduction

What do doctors do? To my children it's simple: I make people better. When I go to work, I attend to sick people and get them back to being well. It's an idea that's admirable for its simplicity and logic. We are either ill or we are well. If we are well, we have no need of doctors. If we are ill, we should ask a doctor for advice so that we can return to health.

And I do manage this kind of thing, but only rarely. I qualified in medicine in 1994, graduating with a list of things that I had been taught I must never forget, such as Cushing's syndrome or osteosarcoma or allergic alveolitis. I had been taught by experts and enthusiasts, all anxious that I should realise the importance of their own specialty and, usually, their pet disease (all specialists have these, though they may not admit it.) Not many of these are common to a GP, although there are certain conditions that I am always anxious to recognise because treatment can make someone genuinely better, and this makes for my joy. Hypothyroidism, for example, classically manifests as weight gain, low mood, dry skin and hair that tends to fall out: if you remember to test for it, you can truly make someone better with a blood test or two, and some cheap thyroid hormone tablets. Depression, too, has to be one of the best things to treat as a doctor; it gives me great satisfaction to see an optimistic, happy person re-emerge from the distressed individual who originally sat down with me.

The problem is that I don't often see, or suspect, Cushing's syndrome, osteosarcoma or allergic alveolitis. The clear-cut diagnosis promised by medical school textbooks rarely transpires. Instead, I see people who have had a dreadful bereavement and whose income support has been stopped, who are in debt and not sleeping, or who are anxious and scared. The textbooks might say that I should consider depression but the new breed of diagnostic questionnaires, which I am strongly encouraged to use if I suspect depression, do not come with the ability to understand why the person is so afraid. Or someone might present with a pain that sometimes comes when they walk, and sometimes doesn't, and which is sometimes below the knee and sometimes above it – yet which matches none of the textbook descriptions of anything easily diagnosable or treatable.

So what do doctors do? As someone who felt she had a vocation to practise medicine, and who spends her days trying to work out how to help people, the truth is difficult to admit. It is that medicine has got its priorities muddled up to such an extent that doctors are capable of harming people just as often – or even more often – as they help them.

How? Side-effects of powerful drugs? Misdiagnosis? Wrong operations, or the wrong leg being removed? All these are possible but, to my mind, none is the biggest issue that we face. Side-effects occur with all drugs and must be weighed up against the benefits. I think doctors have got better at criticising drugs and being rightfully cautious about prescriptions. Misdiagnosis? Diagnosis is just as much of an art as a science and is always going to involve subjectivity and some uncertainty. Wrong operations? Human error can be minimised, but never excluded.

All these things are important, but the biggest change to medicine that has arisen over the course of my career has been the seeming determination of healthcare professionals to bring healthy people into surgeries and clinics, and turn them into patients. I am no longer there to make people better, I am there to find out what risk factors for disease they might have or could have, despite their feeling well and having no complaints at all. Shouldn't general practice be there to deal with people who are in physical or mental pain, who have noticed a worrying lump or who need their diabetes medication adjusted?

Apparently not. Now doctors are there to do cervical smears, to screen for depression, to look for the possible early signs of kidney disease or bowel cancer, to recommend mammography or load people onto weighing scales. Cholesterols, blood pressures and sugar levels are measured millions of times in people who are at low risk of disease. The 'well person' clinic is not a service offered ironically. Doctors have even been known to set up 'well man' clinics in pubs or football stadiums to 'reach out' to people who have no intention of making an appointment. The well are medicine's new domain.

What's the problem with that? Isn't it good that doctors want to prevent illness and disease – isn't this good for patients, who after all do pay for the whole NHS? How does that old Chinese proverb go? The mediocre doctor treats disease, the excellent doctor prevents it.

Unfortunately, I disagree, which is a shame because as a person of enthusiasm and passion, I would enjoy trying to think of ways to get fit and healthy people in to see me in order to spare them an untimely death. I believe in the moral necessity of reducing the burden of ill health among the poorest people in society. If we could deal with both in a medical double whammy, I would happily devote my time to pulling people off the street and into a blood pressure cuff.

But the reality behind prevention is one of medicine's dirty little secrets. The cervical screening programme, for example, manages to create a vast number of cervical smears that are 'borderline' or 'abnormal', causing the need for further testing and enormous anxiety to the women concerned – despite the fact that most changes would revert to normal all by themselves. We look for ways to reduce breast cancer incidence without realising that the biggest problem is the overdiagnosis of cancer on screening mammograms – 'cancer' that was always unlikely to maim or kill. We drag people back and forward to the surgery to monitor weight, cholesterol or blood pressure, overlooking the fact that the biggest influences on health are not medicine but poverty, diet, stress and work. And medicine itself is responsible for creating anxiety, needless diagnoses and pointless to-ing and fro-ing from the surgery. People are becoming patients, and there is a cost involved.

And in the meantime, what happens to the people who are depressed, who have found a lump, or who have what might just be Cushing's disease?

Here is the crunch, the ludicrous inversion of where care is and isn't forthcoming in today's NHS. If there is nothing wrong with you, you will receive personalised letters, glossy leaflets, access to special phone lines and kind encouragement to attend for whatever screening tests the NHS would like to offer you.

If you are ill, however, it is entirely different. For those who are anxious and depressed, the so-called talking therapies can be a useful treatment. Accessing them, however, is often a nightmare. You may be asked to phone a number between certain times. Someone may then phone you back to arrange an assessment appointment. At the assessment appointment, you may be told to make another appointment or you may be placed on a waiting list. While on the waiting list, you may be expected to phone regularly to say that you wish to remain on it. When you finally reach the top, you may be told to phone a certain number between certain times or risk losing your place in the queue altogether.

Doing all this when you are well would perhaps be testing. When you are fragile, vulnerable and distressed, it can become nigh-on impossible. Only the least ill may end up getting any help at all.

That's the paradox that I keep finding within the NHS: if you are ill, you may have to be persistent and determined to get help. GPs have to be persistent too. Yet if you are well, you are at risk of being checked and screened into patienthood, given preventive medication for something you'll never get, or treated for something you haven't got.

This book is my attempt to explain this paradox to people at risk of being turned into patients. It is also a plea to the voters, the administrators and the politicians responsible for the NHS to consider what we are trying to achieve and for whom.

What I'd really like to be able to do is agree with my children. Agree that as a doctor, I at least do my best to make ill people better.

PART ONE

People made into patients

1

To screen or not to screen: first do no harm

Is it possible to be in perfect health? Not any more. The only normal person is one that that hasn't had modern medicine unleashed on them. Take a perfectly well person and run blood tests, scans, X-rays or bowel tests – and there may be a blood level that's above average, a possible hint of a shadow on a scan. Still feeling well, still in perfect health? Alas, our collective love-in with too many medical tests has run away with our common sense and produced a big problem. The screening of people for disease causes enormous problems which don't often get acknowledged – not even to the people having the tests.

This is medical screening in action. Screening tests don't involve people who are ill or have symptoms. First off, if you are ill, you need to be checked out. This is not screening. If you have a lump that worries you, a tendency to collapse without warning, an itch that won't go away or any other complaint about your health, you are symptomatic. Symptoms need sorting. Generally, that means seeing a doctor who will take 'a history', giving you time to describe and explain what is happening. So: 'For the past three months I've had this itching under my skin so bad that I scratch myself until I bleed. I can't think why, but it's worse after a shower.' The doctor asks you questions designed to hone in. Have you been abroad? Anyone else itchy? Anything new you're putting on your skin?

He is then meant to examine you, looking for a rash or evidence of infestation with lice or scabies, or other lovely creatures. The diagnosis may not be definite and tests may be needed to increase the certainty – a skin scraping or maybe a blood sample. Finally, diagnosis is followed by treatment, with follow-up to ensure that all is going to plan and that the side-effects of treatment are not disabling or worse than the condition.

Screening is not about sorting out ill people. Many politicians and, sadly, some people who work in healthcare don't understand this. So, for example, breast screening is offered to women who have no complaints of breast lumps. Depression screening is offered to people who are not complaining of mental ill health. Screening is not about working out what is going on when, for example, a woman complains of chest pain or a man confides that he has suicidal impulses.

The difference is important. I've had angry emails from people telling me that if they hadn't got 'screened' they'd be dead. Often, though, those people had not been screened – they had been diagnosed on the basis of symptoms. It's very different.

So, if you are a man with no complaints about your ability to urinate or copulate, are feeling hearty but decide you'd like a prostate check-up anyway, you are embarking on the process of being screened.

The ethical practice of medicine means being honest about the limitations and potential harms of interventions as well as the benefits. And as for what Hippocrates said...

'First do no harm'

Screening throws Hippocrates out of the window. We have no screening test without side-effects. Harm is inevitable. With any screening programme, the gamble is taken that ultimately, it will cause more good than harm. This is the essence of why screening is difficult and can be summed up in a beautiful and counterintuitive puzzle. Try this:

A disease affects 1% of the population. It is fatal. There is no treatment. The test for this condition is 90% accurate. So if you test positive for the disease, how likely are you to have it?

Most people read this question and say that you are 90% likely to have the dreaded disease, and agree that your priority is now writing your will and working out what your last wishes are. It seems logical: the test is 90% accurate, so that's how likely you are to have the disease.

It's also wrong. The '90% accurate' bit refers to how likely you are *both* to have the disease and test positive for it. So if you have 100 people with the disease, only 90 of them – 90% – will test positive for it.

This is the crunch. If you are being screened for the disease, which only affects 1% of the population, then you only have a risk of 1% of having it.

Let's make the numbers easy. Say we have 1,000 people, and ten of them – 1% – have the disease. If the test is 90% accurate, it will pick up nine of them. One person will test negative even though he has the disease.

But that test is also 90% accurate for the people who *do not* have the disease. This means, that out of the 990 people who don't

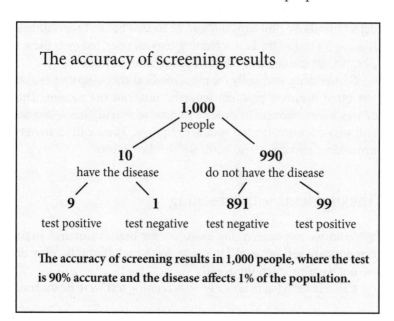

The accuracy of screening results

```
                        1,000
                        people
                   /              \
              10                      990
         have the disease         do not have the disease
          /        \                 /          \
        9            1            891              99
   test positive  test negative  test negative  test positive
```

The accuracy of screening results in 1,000 people, where the test is 90% accurate and the disease affects 1% of the population.

have it, 99 will end up testing positive for a disease they don't have.

So in total, out of that 1,000 people, 99+9 people test positive, 108 in total.

But only nine of those people really do have the disease.

So if you test positive for this disease, your chance is only nine out of 108 that you really do have the disease – about a 10% chance.

The first time I learned about this I remember being very shocked. How could a pretty good test – 90% accurate! – be so rubbish?

It's mainly because the risk of having the disease is still pretty low. If you run a test in someone who has a high risk of having the disease – for example, if you are running the same test in a population where 50 of 100 people have the disease, not one in 100 – the odds of the same test being more accurate will increase. But when we are screening for disease, we are usually looking for things that are relatively rare. Thus starts the difficulty in making sure that testing positive for a disease is a reliable sign that you actually have it.

Certainly there are rare screening tests that are useful, for example the Guthrie test, which is done in newborn babies to detect metabolic problems that can be treated before brain damage is done. It's one of the best screening tests on offer, but even then, a positive test result is only verified in a minority of cases.

Remarkably, and sadly for most medical check-ups, a positive test often means a problem with the test, not the patient. This causes harm because in order to know who truly has a disease and who does not, further tests are required. These can be anxiety provoking, and can cause harm within themselves.

The problems with screening

Why do we not screen, for example, for brain tumours? Brain tumours are serious, and can cause death and disability. Why do we not want to 'catch them early'?

Criteria for what makes a good screening test were established by the World Health Organization in 1968.[1] For example, there is no point screening for a disease for which you don't have a great solution. If you screen for and then find 1,000 cases of an incurable disease, as some brain tumours sadly are, then you haven't helped very much – all you have done is identified some tumours earlier. You could argue that this is a bad thing. It's certainly not useful.

Useful screening means finding an unsuspected disease at a stage where you can treat and, ideally, cure it. A perfect screening

---

WHO definition of screening tests

1. The condition sought should be an important health problem.
2. There should be an accepted treatment for patients with recognized disease.
3. Facilities for diagnosis and treatment should be available.
4. There should be a recognizable latent or early symptomatic stage.
5. There should be a suitable test or examination.
6. The test should be acceptable to the population.
7. The natural history of the condition, including development from latent to declared disease, should be adequately understood.
8. There should be an agreed policy on whom to treat as patients.
9. The cost of case-finding (including diagnosis and treatment of patients diagnosed) should be economically balanced in relation to possible expenditure on medical care as a whole.
10. Case-finding should be a continuing process and not a 'once and for all' project.

Wilson JMG and Jungner G, World Health Organization, Geneva, 1968

---

test would be one that was always right, neither invasive nor unpleasant, with a cure that was always successful and with no side-effects. Welcome to la-la land.

There is no such thing as a perfect screening test – not that you'd know from the sexed-up inducements, incitements and fervour attached to screening in the UK.

The myth of the body MOT

One of the great Harley Street sells is the medical 'check-up'. Even smart people equate our bodies to cars requiring MOTs at least once a year. Competing clinics, many operating in chains, offer testing packages that are described in terms that may seem better suited to first-class airline travel or gym memberships: 'premium', 'ultimate' and, bafflingly, 'ultimate plus'. These check-ups will cost you from hundreds to thousands of pounds and are designed for people who want to 'take control' of their health and won't mind spending a few hundred or thousand pounds for the treat. Prescan, a company working out of Harley Street, says that 'a preventative examination will enable you to find out in time or just to get some certainty regarding your health'.[2] Lifescan has worked 'in partnership' with Tesco Clubcard to offer you a 'check for the very early signs of heart disease, lung cancer, colon cancer, aneurysms and osteoporosis as well as other illnesses'.[3]

Well, we are all at risk of dying. These companies want you to believe that the check-up will heroically save you from death. Either you will be reassured that everything is fine and this knowledge, despite its effect on your bank balance, will cheer and sustain you. Or you will have your cancer or heart disease diagnosed. You have it spotted early. You are still a winner. It may seem as though this is a bet that wins each way. If the test is 'all-clear', then you can feel pleasure and relief. If the test shows a problem, you can feel virtuous in knowing that your proactivity has saved you from your early fate.

Sadly it's not true. We are not cars. The clinics are offering screening tests, which do not obey superficially logical assumptions.

Instead, screening tests are complex and their outcomes are often counter-intuitive.

Still, it's hard to emphasise the absence of evidence when you get tales of salvation through the whole body MOT, such as this, from the front page of the Prescan website:

> 'Prescan's MRI revealed a two inch kidney tumour – if it had been left unchecked my story would have a very different ending!'

Or, from the celebrity-packed Preventicum testimonial webpage:

> 'My check-up was far more thorough than I had anticipated and the doctors detected a brain aneurysm as a result of my MRI scan. This came as a complete shock to say the least. Luckily, thanks to Preventicum, it was detected early enough to be successfully treated and I was back at work less than three months after the surgery. I wholeheartedly recommend having this check-up, whether you have a specific concern or just want to find out how healthy you really are. Preventicum certainly saved my life.'

Magnetic resonance imaging, MRI, and high-resolution CT (computerised tomography) are the best in modern medical imaging. What was a blurry snowstorm 50 years ago is now rendered in three-dimensional digital clarity, shining pictures of kidneys, livers, lungs and brains onto monitors seconds after scanning. Modern equipment is smaller, quieter, and less intimidating. The private check-up sector – and they accept most credit cards – has erupted as these scanners have become cheaper and better in quality.

Scams and scans

The fact that there is so much choice about what kind of deluxe health check to have is a pointer to the problem at the heart of the scanning-on-payment industry. You can have any number of permutations of imaging: a lung check, a colon check, a heart scan, a bone mineral scan, a brain scan or womb or prostate scan. Most companies are keen to stress that they'll make adjustments to pricing structures according to your desire. Hey, it's a customer thing.

These clinics are often owned by medically qualified doctors. Some are not and just have doctors working there. Doctors are required because of the regulation controlling ionising (X-ray) radiation. With doctors on board, the clinics appear more legitimate, honourable and regulated, offering a responsible way to execute your responsibilities to your health, pleasing to the 'self-care' mantra, and, overall, a good way to spend your time and cash.

It would be reasonable, therefore, to expect some evidence supporting this kind of screening. Proof of usefulness that might mean there is a chance that the scans would be better for your health than, say, running away from these clinics at top speed with your cash still in your pocket.

Here's the story of Brian Mulroney, the former Canadian Prime Minister, as told to me by H Gilbert Welch, public heath doctor and author of *Should I be tested for cancer? Maybe not and here's why.*[4]

'In 2005, he went to the doctors for a routine check-up. As part of the check-up, he had a spiral CT scan. It showed two small, but worrisome nodules. He had surgery to have them removed. Post-operatively, he developed pancreatitis – a complication of surgery.'

The nodules, which were on the lung, had been removed, but Mulroney had to be moved into the intensive care unit of the hospital.

'After a month and a half in the hospital, he was discharged to convalesce at home. Then he had to be readmitted a month later to have an operation on a cyst that had developed around his pancreas – a complication of pancreatitis. He was in the hospital another month. Oh, and he didn't even have lung cancer. They were just checking.'[5]

Mulroney had a false positive. His doctors thought he had something seriously wrong – they were probably worried about an early cancer. They acted accordingly, accruing recognised complications of the tests needed to work out if these nodules were cancer or not. Mulroney didn't benefit from the screening – he was harmed by it. Do we know how common this kind of harm is? We don't. Doctors are good at counting benefits of interventions; they are less good at looking for harm.

Take the 'two inch kidney tumour' in the Prescan testimonial above. The test may have flagged up a potential problem, but we don't know whether that cancer was about to cause blood in the urine, which would have naturally – because of symptoms – led to tests to find out why. We don't know if that tumour was likely to cause harm immediately. We know that cancers do not always do what we expect them to. Unless screening like this is tested just like any other medical intervention, you can have no idea if you are helping or harming. This is compounded by 'lead-time bias' (see box below).

What about the brain aneurysm story? It certainly sounds impressive. You may have heard of sudden deaths from bleeds in the brain from these small swellings in the walls of the artery, in perfectly well people, who were otherwise living their lives to the max.

Lead-time bias

A person boards a London-bound train in Glasgow. Another person boards the train in Newcastle. The train crashes in London killing both.

The Glasgow traveller had survived on the train for five hours, the Newcastle passenger for three. Similarly, with lead-time bias, finding a disease earlier can make it seem that the patient survived longer when the end point – time of death – is the same.

Adapted from Professor Mike Baum

On the basis of that particular person's story, it sounds as though screening for brain aneurysms could make for the perfect screening test. It's a condition that you know nothing about until it causes a fatal, or near-fatal, bleed. It can be diagnosed with a scan, meaning no invasive tests need to be done. And as they say, it can be treated.

This neat logic is more like a fairy story.

A paper in the *New England Journal of Medicine* (*NEJM*) in 2010 set out to look at what turns up when scanning the brains of healthy people. More than 2,000 scans were done: they found brain aneurysms in 1.8%, brain infarcts – meaning stroke – in 7.2%, and benign tumours in 1.6%. That's an awful lot of 'normal' people turning out not to be 'normal' at all.

Or are they? The conclusion the study reached was that 'information on the natural course of these lesions is needed to inform clinical management'.[6] Too right! For years doctors had been scanning people with symptoms: people who had symptoms of stroke, problems with vision, blinding headaches. Head scans had been used in these circumstances to work out what the diagnosis was. But scanning healthy, no-symptom people in big numbers simply hadn't been done. We might think we are normal but if we get scanned there is a good chance of finding *something*. Does that make us abnormal?

The Health Technology Assessment Service in Canada examined all the evidence relating to screening for these aneurysms in 2010.[7] It agreed that about 2% of perfectly well people had an aneurysm sitting in their brain that they knew nothing about – no symptoms, feeling perfectly well. Clearly, 2% of the population don't annually rupture a brain aneurysm – the figure is more like 0.01%.[8] The Service assessed the existing evidence and decided that there wasn't enough to recommend screening. It went even further. It is known that people who have a family history of a brain aneurysm are at an increased risk of having one too. Doesn't it make sense to screen for it in this group of people who are at higher risk of having a brain aneurysm? No, the Service found: 'Screening for unruptured intracranial aneurysms in high-risk populations is of uncertain value.'

Why is this? The treatment for unruptured aneurysms involves placing a clip or a coil inside or around the swelling in order to reduce it. This is usually done via a wire passed through an artery, via the groin. Operations in the blood vessels of the brain should not be undertaken lightly. In 1998 the *NEJM* had published a study following up patients with unruptured brain aneurysms and plotting what happened when either leaving them alone or operating on them.[8] If the person had never had a bleed from the brain, and had a small aneurysm, the risk of a bleed was 0.05%, or one in 2,000, per year. The study found that the risks of treatment were higher than previously stated, and the risks of having an aneurysm were lower than previously stated. It concluded that 'It appears unlikely that surgery will reduce the rates of disability and death in patients with unruptured intracranial aneurysms smaller than 10mm in diameter and no history of subarachnoid haemorrhage.' Even for larger aneurysms, there was no clear answer on what to do, because of the risks of operating. The researchers were concerned that the harm of operating was more than the harm of leaving the aneurysm alone. Perhaps if treatment gets even safer, or if imaging studies can recognise riskier aneurysms, the balance of risks might change. Even then, there will be pros and cons to consider.

So an alternative version of that Preventicum testimonial might be: 'I had a scan that I didn't need and had treatment that may or may not have saved my life. Certainly there's no evidence that I spent a few hundred quid on something that did me good. That aneurysm may never have ruptured and the treatment I received could have caused me greater damage. I was lucky it didn't.'

And of course, dead or damaged patients are less able to give their view on the services of private screening clinics to others. Damaged patients may not know that theirs was an avoidable harm.

We are sold screening MOTs as though there were no downside to consider. The adverts from Lifescan picture frolicking couples fizzing with energy as they leap up to claim 'we've been checked!' Preventicum's website boasts that the company offers 'the most advanced and safest health assessments in Europe'. Do any of these adverts adequately reflect the unknowns, the uncertainty and the problems associated with screening well people? Unfortunately not. The evidence is lacking.

More ain't more

Scans aren't the only tests on offer to well people. BUPA offers 'check-ups' ranging from 'core' to 'advanced' and 'complete'. It also has 'supplementary health checks' including 'breast health' and 'coronary health'. The company's 'complete' check offers a 'prostate check' for men over 50, as well as 34 other tests, including those for thyroid conditions and a 'gout test'.[9]

BUPA lists its various options by comparing the duration of the appointment, the consultation time with the doctor the and number of tests and measures.

Let us break this down. How useful is having a test for gout when you are entirely well?

BUPA is talking about a 'uric acid' blood test. Uric acid is a byproduct of muscle breakdown. We eat protein in our diets. Uric acid can be raised when we take 'water tablets' or diuretics for blood pressure or to treat excess fluid in the body.

Uric acid can be slightly raised in people in these categories but it doesn't mean they have gout. No – gout, that ancient, medieval condition where urate crystals gather in a joint causing redness and pain, is a clinical diagnosis. It is not diagnosed by a blood test. It is diagnosed when a person says 'my toe is red and inflamed. It's so sore that even a bedsheet on top is agony.' The doctor examines the toe and suspects gout. If the diagnosis is uncertain, a needle can retrieve fluid within the joint, which is inspected microscopically for the tell-tale uric crystals. And all this time the urate level in your blood can be *entirely normal.*

Uric acid levels in blood are not a test for gout. So what if your urate level is slightly high and your toes are not painful and your joints are all normal? You don't have gout, you have a slightly raised uric acid level. It's a very different thing.

If a patient has what looks like gout, measuring uric acid immediately can be misleading, because it can be low during the acute attack. Even if someone has one attack of gout, we wouldn't automatically put him on uric acid-lowering drugs because these potentially have side-effects, and need to be taken long term to work.

Thus, uric acid is not a useful measurement for well people.

It gets worse. How useful is a set of liver function tests in a perfectly well person looking for a bit of a check-up? These tests measure the levels of liver enzymes. You can have liver failure or cirrhosis and these results can be normal. You can be drinking to excess every day of the week and these results can be normal. A study a few years ago looked at people with cancer that had spread to their livers and how frequent abnormal liver function tests were in this group. One-third were completely normal.[10]

Liver function tests (LFTs) were not designed to soothe our conscience about how much we drink or eat. If you are drinking too much, you are drinking too much. If you are eating too much rubbishy food, your liver tests may be normal, but you are still eating too much rubbishy food. A normal set of LFTs proves nothing. If hepatitis is suspected, or a gallstone, then yes, LFTs can be useful. But they are not diagnostic tests – abnormal LFTs may mean many things, from hepatitis to the effects of an overdose of paracetamol to an illness that has nothing much to do with the liver at all. Liver test results need to be tied in with the clinical picture. For example, you would suspect acute hepatitis in a person who was vomiting, fevered and jaundiced; liver tests would be one factor, and not the only factor, in making the diagnosis.

LFTs, like blood urate, are of questionable value in perfectly well people. They can't reliably detect people in trouble, nor can they reassure healthy people that their lifestyle is suiting them well. They aren't good screening tests.

Screening tests, you'll remember, are tests to be done when attempting to diagnose an unsuspected disease at an earlier stage to allow for advantageous treatment. What should be a careful, well-thought out diagnostic process has mutated into a bludgeoning battle axe – an instrument so crude it doesn't really know what it is testing for.

Do we even know that much about LFT readings in normal people? Between 1% and 9% of healthy 'normal' people have 'abnormal' results.[11]

Are they even 'abnormal'? The point at which 'normal' ends and 'abnormal' begins is not a straightforward boundary when it comes to biochemical – and many other – tests. Most of the numbers attached to laboratories' 'normal/abnormal' results are based on reference ranges. These are typically collections of data from normal volunteers. Yet there are major biases even here. For example, one collection of results contained only young men – no women, older people, or variations in ethnic group.[12] Older people are known to have variations for some biochemical tests that are quite normal for them although they are outside 'normal' parameters for younger people.

The standard way of calculating when a biochemical result becomes abnormal is simply numerical. Normal human values generally follow a 'bell curve' – a graph shaped like a bell. More normal results are pitched in the middle, falling away to fewer as you go out from the middle to the sides. In the mathematical description of 'normal' it is automatically accepted that many 'normal' results will sit outside the majority values.

There are other factors too. The same person who has ten different normal LFTs taken over a week will be unlikely to score exactly the same in each test. Then there is machine variability. The equipment laboratories use to generate test results will not always generate two identical readings on a single sample of blood.

If you are trying to decide what 'normal' is, you may find it difficult. So how do you start to decide if a LFT measurement taken as part of a check-up is a good idea when it's hard enough deciding where 'normal' starts and ends?

Wouldn't you want to know what you're getting into before you have the test? You might even hope to see BUPA and others offering a little caveat saying that a batch of LFTs as a 'check-up' isn't a validated screening test. If you've been enticed by it and

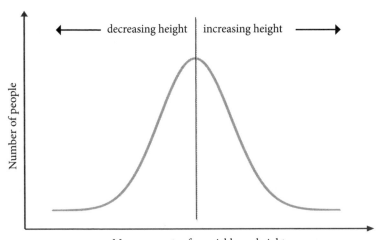

Measurements of a variable, eg height

The bell curve of 'normal' distribution values.

want it, customer, you can buy it. But pause to consider: is that freedom as a customer to wave your cash around actually doing you any favours?

Genes and screens

Do you remember where you were when it was announced that the human genome had been mapped in its entirety, with each of the three billion bases that make up our genetic code identified? Neither do I; but it was in 2000 and it was a big story. It was going to be the end of disease, the beginning of breakthroughs that were going to transform healthcare and humanity itself.

Well, it hasn't happened so far. What we do have though is an eager coterie of companies offering genetic screens. It's easy to spend upwards of £1,000 on having your genes mapped. Typical websites offer 'empowerment' and have pictures of lithe young women riding bicycles, with messages like: 'Live life to the fullest'.

Most of these companies offer to check for genetic 'risk factors'. As a doctor, I'm more used to dealing with genetic diseases – that is, disorders that are passed by single or groups of genes. Examples include Huntington's disease, a disorder of movement, or cystic fibrosis. Genetic screening as offered by commercial companies mainly isn't concerned with these types of disorders. Instead, they are more concerned with genetic risk factors.

It's a little bit of déjà vu. We seem to have sidled into another arena of the indefinite, the uncertain and the vague.

Consider the 'Premium Female Gene' screen from the trendily lower-case 'genetichealth'. This promises to tell you:

'The advantages and disadvantages of hormone replacement therapy by considering your genetic predisposition to: breast cancer, bone metabolism, thrombosis, cancer and long-term exposure to estrogens.'

It goes on:

'With this dynamic information your doctor can:
- Give advice specifically tailored to you for disease prevention and longevity
- Choose for you a customized HRT treatment or other hormone treatment that suits you best, thus reducing harmful side-effects
- Advise you on the small but specific changes that you can make in your lifestyle that will greatly affect your health and happiness.'[13]

I find this rather amazing. A genetic screen that can make you *happier*?

Let us rewind. What evidence do we have for any of this? What long-term, randomised controlled trials (RCTs) have been done showing us that a genetic screening will result in happier lives or lives with less disease or death?

It's well known that some female diseases, such as breast cancer or ovarian cancer, can have genetic links, although around 95% of breast cancers don't.[14] Where there is a suspected genetic pattern within a family, NHS genetics clinics are geared up to discuss testing its implications. It is an easy test to do – but shouldn't be done lightly.

Randomised controlled trial (RCT)

How do patients and doctors know what treatments or interventions work? Is the treatment good, is it harmful, or have people got better not because of a treatment but because they were going to anyway?

The gold standard is a placebo controlled randomised controlled trial, 'blinded' so that neither doctor nor patient knows who is getting which intervention.

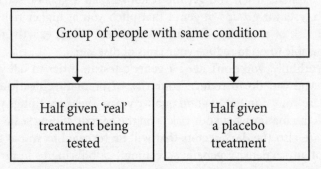

Did they get better, worse, or stay the same? Outcomes of treatments are measured and compared.

Why not instant testing? Even when women have a laboratory-proven genetic disorder that carries a high risk of ovarian or breast cancer, there is debate about how useful frequent and/or early screening is. Mammography, for all its faults as a screening test in any circumstances, is especially poor for identifying cancer in the younger, premenopausal breast. Ultrasound is known to be too error-prone to be useful. For women at high or very high risk of breast cancer, through, for example, the *BRCA* or *TP53* genetic mutations, annual MRI scan surveillance is now offered.[15] However, there is still debate about how successful this will be.[16] Very high risk women may consider mastectomy even when there is no cancer in the breast. It's already known that women at ordinary risk of ovarian cancer don't benefit from screening for it.[17] For women at high risk of ovarian cancer, even this is currently only done as part of a clinical trial because it isn't clear that it can reduce deaths from ovarian cancer.[18]

And this is people with known, definite, genetic disorders that give a 'yes' or 'no' answer – for example, whether or not you have the *BRAC* group of genes that make you more prone to certain types of cancer. Commercial screening companies aren't usually interested in clear genetic abnormalities with one or two clear genetic changes, but instead in groups of genes that may be more likely to be associated with vascular disease or other illnesses. So what happens when you get the result of such a 'genetic screen', which tests for groups of genes that pitch you at higher risk or lower risk of a variety of vaguer diagnoses? What, exactly, will you be able to do to reduce your risks of disease?

Truthfully, you don't need a genetic test in order to tell you what you can do to reduce your risk of premature death and increase your number of good quality years. These are things you can do no matter what your risk is on the genetic sliding scale yet they are also the dark secrets that will be revealed to you at the end of any expensive genetic screening test offering to improve your life. And what are these medical mysteries?

For free: don't smoke. Don't drink excessively, and not every day. Eat a wide variety of foods, mainly fruits and vegetables. Exercise daily, and if you can, make it sociable. Have a job you like. See people and do things you enjoy. Stay reasonably trim. And don't be poor.

This, cunningly, is exactly the same advice that I would give anyone who hasn't had a genetic screen done.

The cautious customer might just be asking what the genetic screen can actually help with, given that the advice, whether screened or unscreened, remains the same.

The even more cautious customer might ask what the point of splashing out on the same outcome might be – and whether or not there could be harm in the advice given out by clinics anxious to dispel the illusion that there isn't much point to their service.

Take for example a piece by Jonathan Margolis, writing in the

Financial Times' How to Spend It supplement about his own genetic screen. He concludes that his daughters may have a small increase in risk in breast cancer. 'Both daughters, while not pleased about this, now at least feel themselves duly alerted and vigilant.'[19]

What a lovely gift from your dad. We don't even have evidence, believe it or not, that telling women to check their breasts regularly is a useful way to prevent deaths from breast cancer (and we'll discuss this in more detail later). We have no evidence that screening younger women does more good than harm. We do know that having chronic anxiety or depression is likely to be bad for you.[20] How has dad helped by obtaining this information?

Well, we could tell you to take regular exercise, avoid excessive alcohol, excessive weight, to eat a diet rich in fruit and vegetables . . . all of which we know to be good for health – yes, exactly the same advice we would give you anyway.

Supposing a woman were to find out that her risk of breast cancer was lower than average. What then? Would she ignore a breast lump, thinking it was less likely to be a cancer? Would she drink or smoke more, thinking she was more likely, with her advantageous genetic code, to get away with it? Such behaviour might bring her breast cancer risk back up to average and may simply increase the risks of vascular or other illnesses.

What we need is a big study that asks these questions about harms as well as benefits. It hasn't been done. Instead, genetic screening is touted as a simple, fast breakthrough when the results are anything but.

Why we need to do it with evidence

You've seen those news reports that begin: 'Medical research shows . . .' Alas, 'medical research' is a tangled mess of studies that don't need to be done, studies that are too small or badly designed to be of any use, and studies that fail to address genuinely important questions. Medical research is not uniformly reliable. More on this later but for now, as a GP, I know that many specialist doctors believe that their area of expertise is the one that is undervalued, underfunded and inadequately recognised by GPs, patients and politicians. This is one of the reasons why 'expert opinion' as a form of evidence is considered by many to be the lowest and least reliable of all the types of evidence available.[21] (See diagram on opposite page.)

We are all fallible humans, shaped by the uniqueness of our experience. If I particularly remember the tragedy of a young patient dying of lung cancer (and I do), I may, for months afterwards, be overanxious about any vaguely unwell, similarly aged patient. Were I able to rationalise and use logic and statistics to guide me rather than my simmering anxiety about a horrible (but extremely remote) chance of a repeat case, it would help me to be a more accurate clinician. I know that lung cancer in under 35 year olds is rare. Yet my worrying nature may trump my knowledge, if I don't keep it in check. I may end up ordering X-rays on everyone – over-investigating – if I don't keep a handle on the scientific evidence for what I'm doing.

The use of evidence is crucial to medical professionalism. Without evidence, I would be simply making it up as I went along. The use of evidence in medicine has not been consistent. For example, a US advert from 1949 starts like this:

'Time out for many men of medicine usually means just long enough to enjoy a cigarette. And because they know what a pleasure it is to smoke a mild good tasting cigarette, they're particular about the brand they choose. In a repeated national survey, doctors in all branches of medicine, in all parts of the country were asked "What cigarette do you smoke, doctor?" Once again, the brand named most was Camel.'[22]

The advert showed a handsome male doctor puffing all over his pretty nurse. It took several decades, many large studies and an awful lot of bickering before doctors eventually accepted that smoking didn't provide 'your throat protection against irritation against cough'[23] but instead provided mouth cancer, throat cancer and lung cancer. The doctors were happy to be used in advertising

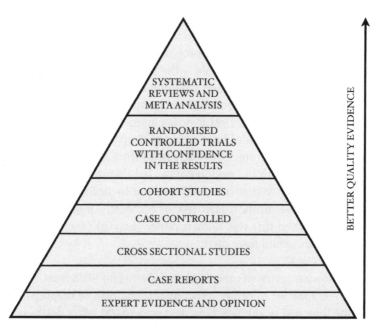

The hierarchy of the quality of evidence.

photographs to sell cigarettes because they simply believed their own opinion.

Or what about Dr Benjamin Spock? An avowed childcare guru, he wrote *Baby and Child Care*, which sold more than 50 million copies and was translated into 39 languages – supposedly 'second in sales only to the bible'.[24] One edition was produced for use 'under the National Health Service'. He told readers, in his 1958 edition, that:

> 'There are two disadvantages to a baby's sleeping on his back. If he vomits, he is more likely to choke on the vomitus. Also, he tends to keep his head turned toward the same side – usually toward the centre of the room. This may flatten that side of his head. . . . I think it is preferable to accustom a child to sleeping on his stomach from the start if he was willing.'[25]

This became the norm. Putting your newborn to sleep on their stomach was the right thing to do. By 1970 there was evidence that putting children to sleep in this way raised the risk of sudden infant death syndrome, or SIDS. No one paid much heed to what the evidence said – the power of conventional and popular 'wisdom' outweighed anything else.

By the time formal 'Back to Sleep' campaigns were launched by the UK government in 1991,[26] now persuaded that the evidence showed that babies should not be put to sleep on their fronts, huge damage had been done. One study from the Centre of Evidence-Based Child Health in London concluded that in 1970, there was adequate evidence that if a child was put to sleep on his or her front, there was an increased risk of cot death. If attention had been paid when this was known rather than 20 years later then fewer babies would have died:

> 'Systematic review of preventable risk factors for SIDS from 1970 would have led to earlier recognition of the risks of sleeping on the front and might have prevented over 10,000 infant deaths in the UK and at least 50,000 in Europe, the USA, and Australasia.'[27]

I find this quite frightening. One has to accept the possibility that what seems logical and useful may even have harmful effects.

Ten years ago, if you had a serious head injury and you were taken to hospital, you may have been given a dose of steroids. The rationale was simple: head injuries can kill, often because the injury causes brain swelling. This swelling is damaging to the extent that it can cause death rather than the initial head injury.

Steroids are fantastic at reducing swelling in most parts of the body, from joints to bowels to lungs. It was quite logical, then, to use steroids in people who had a severe head injury in order to prevent or treat brain injury. Wasn't it?

Steroids were used in head injury for more than a decade before scientists and doctors admitted that they actually didn't know if they were harmful or helpful. To ask this question requires tremendous courage: not only do you have to question yourself, but also the care you and your colleagues have given to patients already. Do you really want to know that you have harmed the patients you thought you were helping?

The trial set up to answer this fundamental question was the CRASH trial. It randomly selected patients with serious head injury either to receive steroids or not. When the results came in, it was found that steroids were neither effective nor neutral. They were actively harmful to the extent that if you were given them, you were more likely to die.[28] It was calculated that around 10,000 patients would not have died had this research been done sooner and the use of steroids stopped in these circumstances.[29]

The logic and good intentions that fuelled the prescriptions for steroids in head injury were not enough. This is a horribly hard lesson.

The top of the pyramid: why believe a Cochrane review?

Cochrane reviews, compared to other medical reports, can appear quite odd. Superficially, they appear fairly boring – go to the Cochrane Library and you will see thousands of reviews, short conclusions, and lots of plain text. But these are among the most powerful tools in medicine. It's better not to rely on one small study – it's more reliable to repeat studies, to ensure that the findings are real and not down to chance. This helps to ensure that uncertainties about the results are reduced as far as possible. Cochrane reviews are not ordinary 'reviews' of the evidence. Doing a quick sift through a few easily reachable papers sitting at the top of your desk is not quite Cochrane.

Instead, the goal of a Cochrane review is to ask a clear question. For example, what is the safest sleeping position for babies? Do multivitamins lengthen life in adults? Does flu vaccination stop pneumonia? Does breast screening reduce deaths?

These may sound like boring, straightforward questions, which you might have hoped medicine had already asked by now. Sadly, the best questions are not always the ones that research answers and no wonder, with an agenda dictated in the main by pharmaceutical companies. The research priorities of patients and front line doctors and nurses are rarely addressed. It's often easier to rely on the 'latest' evidence – far easier than studying dusty archived journals in the cellar of a library. Yet these may hold a better quality of answer.

Cochrane reviews take account of all evidence, old or new, far or near. Again, that sounds rather simple, doesn't it: why on earth wouldn't you want to know about *all* the evidence? Alas, and alas again. The ideal would be this: patients, doctors and researchers work out what they want to know. Researchers tell us what we already know, and where the gaps are. Everyone works together to answer the pertinent questions. Researchers analyse the data and tell us what we now know. Then all work together again to implement the findings.

This model of research is tantalisingly straightforward but so groundbreaking that it's hardly ever done — of which more later. What we know is that there are troves of medical research that never see the light of day. Some researchers say that it's hard to get things published in the big-name journals, but in the end, anyone can publish anything on the internet.

Yet researchers don't make use of it. We know that much research sits gathering dust in a filing cabinet. Some estimates say one in three studies never make it into full daylight.[30] We know that pharmaceutical companies routinely bury research that they don't like (one honourable exception is GlaxoSmithKline, which announced it would publish trial data of marketed products in 1995.)[31,32] The globally bestselling anti-inflammatory drug, Vioxx (rofecoxib), was estimated to have been prescribed to 80 million people before being withdrawn from sale in 2004 due to the risk of heart attack or stroke. In 2005, the *NEJM* published an 'expression of concern' about favourable data it published about the drug – in 2000. It appeared that some of the researchers knew about heart attacks in patients on rofecoxib but did not include them in the results that were published.[33]

Unless you have all the data, you don't know what you don't know. This has the potential to harm and kill patients.

Cochrane reviewers scrape the barrel. They hand-search journals and write to people they know have an interest in the subject for any unpublished research they might have stuffed in a drawer. They contact pharmaceutical companies to ask for data. They do lots of tedious legwork. They do this in order to get as good and as fair an answer to a question as possible. Sure, people can still withhold data from you: but Cochrane researchers look as hard as they can.

That's why I believe Cochrane reviews to be reliable: they haven't just chosen to look for research that was easy to find. They have looked for all of it.

The bottom line is that we cannot afford to base medical practice on opinion. The need for evidence is overwhelming. Doctors shouldn't go around telling people to take up smoking in order to clear their throats, or put their baby to sleep on their front just because they think they are right. Doctors need to put opinions to one side and examine research, without bias, to see what it says, no matter how much pride we have to swallow. Otherwise, we do harm – we may even cause death.

2

The business of cardiovascular risk

The Labour Party manifesto in 2010 promised 'preventative health-care routine check-ups for all those aged over 40 years'.[1] They weren't elected, but the Scottish Government announced the same year that 'face to face universal health checks for all Scots aged 40-74' were to be implemented 'for all individuals . . . not just those believed to be at risk.'[2] Additionally, the Department of Health has pledged to offer all adults aged between 40-74 in England a 'health check'.[3]

Locating, examining and testing, explaining, treating and monitoring cardiovascular risk makes up a large chunk of general practice and nursing time within the NHS. It is also big business on the high street. The big idea is that we can calculate future risk of vascular disease based on current measurements, like blood pressure, and intervene to prevent vascular damage such as heart attacks, strokes, ministrokes and kidney damage.

For the person without known vascular disease, a cardiovascular risk assessment is complex; so, too, are the decisions that follow the results. The modern approach to cardiovascular risk has moved on from advising the cessation of smoking, plenty of exercise, and fruit and vegetables. The modern drive is to manage cholesterol levels, blood pressures and, in the private sector, to scan our arteries and pronounce on their fitness. But does all this make us healthier?

What's your cholesterol?

Our obsession with cholesterol cardiac risk assessment is relatively recent. One of the perks of working in the coronary care unit as a junior doctor was, because you weren't allowed to leave the unit, you could phone the canteen and order whatever food you liked for lunch. The canteen staff surpassed themselves and I used to feast on my tray of cheesecake and chips while writing up notes. Delicious. I was learning lots, I was a useful cog in a busy ward: I loved it.

My feast would be interrupted occasionally by a cardiologist, who would appear, stethoscope in hand, frown at my lunch and ask me: wasn't I worried about my cholesterol?

In 1995, when this regular scene of debauched lunch took place, cholesterol was something that you wanted below six (mmol/l), preferably. Sometime in the next couple of years I was lectured to and told that below five was much better. Then the same cardiologist, speaking at a meeting a few years after that, told us all quite plainly: no matter what your cholesterol is, it would be better if it were lower.

Cholesterol is the alleged devil in the arteries of the western world. To exorcise it, you can start with getting your cholesterol tested at any private clinics offering screenings, your local GP or pharmacy counter. I even came across a margarine manufacturer offering fingerprick cholesterol tests at an agricultural fair.

High cholesterol – with the exception of the uncommon very high cholesterols found in some genetic conditions – is not a disease. It's just a risk factor for vascular disease – heart attacks, angina, strokes, TIA (transient ischaemic attacks or mini-strokes), some types of kidney disease and peripheral vascular disease – when the blood circulation to the feet starts to fail. Vascular disease means, essentially, that arteries are inefficient and unable to transport blood in the required quantity. This leads to supply problems in the heart or brain. There are loads of large studies backing up the assertion that cholesterol is a risk factor: people who have higher cholesterol have a higher chance of a heart attack or stroke. But there are many other risk factors for vascular disease: your family history, your smoking habits, your body shape and your exercise regime and diet. It just so happens that cholesterol is easy to measure and we have medication capable of reducing it.

The upshot is that testing and treating for cholesterol levels now means that around one in three adults over 45 takes one of the family of cholesterol-lowering statin drugs.[4] That's upwards of 7 million people in the UK. Back when I was drinking coffee and eating muffins in the coronary care unit, statins were mainly for people who had had a heart attack. Later on, when I was being lectured at and taught to get those cholesterols down, it wasn't just people who already had a problem who were being prescribed them. It was people who were well: people who were just 'at risk' of a heart attack or stroke. That's all of us, basically.

Since then, we have kept lowering the threshold at which we're willing to start prescribing statins. How good are statins at preventing heart attacks and strokes? It's incredibly easy to express the same numbers in a way that is designed either to reassure or scare.

This is important to bear in mind when daily news reports insist that too many people are being killed or disabled by heart disease and stroke. 'Doing something' is active, measurable, visible and positive; not prescribing statins or not taking them might be seen as weak, passive – or even negligent.

So if doctors, by merely signing a bit of paper, can issue a prescription and stop those strokes or heart attacks from happening, why wouldn't they? Wouldn't it be a dereliction of duty if they didn't?

I won't answer that now. But I will try to be neutral with the numbers so that at least you can decide for yourself.

Let's take a 60-year-old, non-smoking white woman, living in Glasgow, with a cholesterol of eight, HDL (high density lipoprotein, which is the 'good', or favourable cholesterol) 2, a blood pressure of 160/85, a weight of 100kgs and a height of 160cm. Her risk of developing heart disease, a stroke or a TIA in the next ten years is eight in 100. Her risk of developing diabetes is 18 in 100.

If she takes a statin, there is no change to her risk of diabetes. If she keeps taking it for ten years, her risk of developing cardiovascular disease falls to six in 100.

Let's change that to a male, same details otherwise. His risk of a heart attack or other vascular disease is 14 in 100 over ten years; his risk of diabetes is 25 in 100.

Taking a statin will reduce his risk of cardiovascular disease to 11 per 100 over that ten years; his risk of diabetes is unchanged.

There are various other calculators – like the Joint British Societies Cardiac Risk Assessor – where you can enter different blood pressures, cholesterols, weights and smoking habits until you are thoroughly bored. There is no consensus in the UK as to which risk calculator is the best. Since deprivation and ethnicity are risk factors, and many calculators don't include these, if you are either Asian or living in a deprived area, a calculator that doesn't take this into account is likely to underestimate your risk.

So why are the risk calculators different? No matter the statistical skill that goes into working out the sums, any calculator is only as good as the evidence it's based on. The town of Framingham, Massachusetts has been a rich source of data. Long-term studies were begun there in 1948 to study risk

---

Relative / absolute risk

Relative risk – This is always expressed as a risk relative to something else.

Absolute risk – This is usually expressed as a number out of 100 or 1,000.

For example: a drug that reduces the risk of a heart attack from 2 in 100 to 1 in 100. This can be said to cut the risk of heart attack by 50% (relative risk) or from 2 in 100 to 1 in 100 (absolute risk).

factors for cardiovascular disease. These have been enormously influential; yet it is a single town with mainly white inhabitants. The data gathered from this town have resulted in the widely used Framingham Cardiac Risk Score Calculator and permeated most other risk calculators used. There have been many other large-scale studies apart from this. How on earth do you make sense of different results from different places at different times?

An attempt was made to combine high-quality trial results, in the form of a meta-analysis, published in the *Lancet* in 2005. The idea with a meta-analysis is that by making studies larger by combining data, you get greater precision, which reduces the play of chance in producing the results. The researchers looked at 14 randomised trials of statins, which contained just over 90,000 participants. The *Lancet* meta-analysis found that:

> 'There was a 12% proportional reduction in all-cause mortality per mmol/l reduction in LDL cholesterol. This reflected a 19% reduction in coronary mortality. . .'[5]

Which is relative risk. Adding up all the 'major vascular events' there is a difference between the control group and the statin groups of 17.8% versus 14.1% – a difference in absolute risk of 3.7%. The difference between deaths related to cardiovascular disease is smaller: statins can reduce this, the study found, from 4.4% to 3.4%.

That's a difference of 1%.

The side-effects of statin tablets make up a long list – including headaches, rashes and nausea. The most frequent is muscle aches. For some people, this will be a minor irritation; for others, it will be bad enough to make them stop running or dancing or swimming. It's the kind of adverse effect that can start dominoes falling.

I suspect that it is not just doctors who minimise the meaning of 'side-effects'. Your attitude to risk – whether or not you are keen to lower every risk possible, no matter what the cost – may influence your behaviour when faced with complex equations involving benefits versus adverse effects.

Statins in real life

This lady whose doctor encourages her to start a statin is a dancer. The ballroom classes she goes to are also attended by her friends. Tuesday afternoons are her favourite times and her friends know that if she is absent, they had better check on her. She meets them for lunch beforehand and enjoys being included in the social group. The dancing keeps her nimble, balanced and her spirits alive.

She starts a statin. She gets stiff and sore. She tells her friends she is not coming this week – and then the next week, and then the next. She misses her Tuesday afternoons, and after a few months, her friends assume she is not coming back. She is terrified of stopping the tablets, lest a stroke or heart attack strike, but is so achey that getting to the local shops feels like an expedition to Everest. She stops going out, becomes isolated and lonely and has a fall at home. Her confidence evaporates. She has lowered her risk of a vascular problem, true, but she has also had serious adverse effects.

The issue is, surely, how to get that perspective on risk right. It's not good being told that your risk of death can fall by 12% if you take a statin (the relative risk) when that figure is really only 1% (the absolute risk).

Another meta-analysis published in the *Archives of Internal Medicine* in 2006 found no difference in death rates when well people (who hadn't previously had a heart attack, stroke or other vascular problem) took statins compared to those who didn't. In low-risk patients, 133 patients had to be treated for over four years to prevent major cardiovascular events (heart attacks or strokes.) For medium-risk patients, the number is 61; for high-risk patients, 40 are treated to stop one vascular event.[6] Sure, there's a difference; sure, something is happening. But we need to keep it in perspective. The price of avoiding one heart attack or stroke is that an awful lot of other people need to be treated who will never get any benefit from taking the tablets.

These tablets save lives – but the life they save will probably not be yours.

Diabetes and statins

Muscle pains are common side-effects of statins but there are less common effects too. One is rhabdomyolysis, which is not just a muscle ache but muscle breakdown, which in its most serious form causes kidney injury. This is very rare, happening in about one in 20,000 people taking statins.[7]

Somewhere between very rare and rare is the development of diabetes. Diabetes is generally either Type 1 or Type 2. In the first, there is a lack of insulin being made in the body so the person generally needs to take insulin for treatment. In the second type, the body is producing its quota of insulin, but there isn't quite enough of it to go round. The reason is usually that the person is too large for the amount of insulin they produce.

A diagnosis of diabetes, in combination with other risk factors for vascular disease, isn't usually great news. It can certainly be treated and controlled. However, diabetes tends to aggravate other risk factors and heighten them. Among the biggest combined risk is diabetes with smoking.

So what if one of the side-effects of statins was to induce diabetes? It would be rather ironic, given that the statins are meant to protect you from vascular risk, not increase it.

Yet this was the conclusion from one large meta-analysis. In total, these studies contained more than 90,000 participants. They found that for every 255 patients treated with a statin for four years, there was one extra case of diabetes.[8]

A small absolute risk, indeed. But we have now more than seven million people taking statins in the UK. So that adds up to 27,450 extra cases of diabetes in the UK per four years *caused by statins*. This is both an unexpected and an 'unintended adverse effect' and the advice of the researchers (and many of the trials within this meta-analysis were funded by several pharmaceutical companies) was that we should not change our prescriptions of statins based on this study.

But if I were a patient, making a choice about whether to take a statin or not, I think I'd want to know about such potential downsides.

Statins and women

Here's a classic mistake. From a paper in *Clinical Cardiology* in 2008:

> 'Many women, however, need pharmacotherapy to control their hypertension, dyslipidaemia, and diabetes to levels required for decreasing risk. New findings from clinical trials featuring women may enhance their CHD prediction and treatment. However, high coronary risk in many women continues to be under-recognised, and women remain under-treated with statins and other therapeutic agents.'[9]

The writers' logical arc goes like this: women are dying from heart disease. Women have high levels of risk for heart disease. Therefore, you can prevent disease by preventive statin treatment.

Do we know this for sure?

For many years women have been assumed to be the same as men, at least when it comes to clinical trials. Men, very often white men, have been studied, and the results rolled out to every section of the population – women, older people, often children, and every ethnic group – without an intake of breath or the question: will that still work?

It might, and it might not. It can't be assumed that the effect of blood pressure medicine in Caucasian men is the same as in African American women. Genes can mean all kinds of things are different – from the amount of enzymes that digest the medication in question to the distribution of fat under our skins. Older people often have different metabolisms, which can mean that drugs can hang around the body for longer. The application of research done in a fine sliver of the population to everyone else is hazardous.

So what about women taking statins for primary prevention of heart attacks and stroke? Up until 2010, there was no evidence that women with no previous cardiovascular problems did better with statins than without. No trial had shown that women reduced their mortality rates by taking a cholesterol-lowering drug as opposed to placebo. In 2007, in the *Lancet*, two brave North American doctors, noting that 36 million Americans were recommended to take statins, analysed the available data on statins in women. They pooled results from eight large randomised trials comparing statins with placebo and concluded that:

'Statins did not reduce total coronary heart disease events in 10,990 women in these primary prevention trials . . . our analysis suggests that lipid-lowering statins should not be prescribed for true primary prevention in women of any age.'[10]

However, in the journal *Circulation*, in 2010, there was great excitement when we were told that the 'numbers were in' with respect to women. This research team set about doing two things: one was a trial using a statin in women, the other was (another) meta-analysis.

This statin trial, named JUPITER, contained 6,801 women over 60 without previous heart attack or stroke who had higher levels of a blood protein called CRP, which is thought to be raised in people at higher risk of vascular disease. I'm going to ignore all the fluff in the paper comparing deaths from heart attacks or stroke or blood clots and just go for the biggie – all-cause mortality. Total deaths. In the statin group, there were 60 deaths out of 3,426 women. In the control group, there were 77 deaths out of 3,375 women. That's a death rate of 1.75% on statins versus 2.28% not on statins. And in fact, the 'p-value' for these results was 0.12. P-values are used to describe how sure we can be that a

What are p-values?

p-values are measures of confidence in statistical results. There is no tipping point when a p-value suddenly means that a study is reliable.

The standard in medical research is that when a p-value is 0.05 or less, then the result is regarded as 'significant' or unlikely to be due to chance. There is, though, a 1 in 20 chance that the result is due to chance. If the p-value obtained is greater than the magic 0.05, the result is regarded as insignificant, and not reliable.

High p-values mean that it's too risky to believe the result – a chance result becomes hazardously plausible.

You can see that this is a line drawn in the sand; there is nothing special about 1 in 20 other than it's accepted in medical journals through convention. This also means that 1 in 20 papers concluding that something works because the p value is 0.05 are going to be wrong; that result was down to chance alone.

result is not due to luck alone. A high p-value means we are not confident, a low value means that we are more confident.

Here, in the JUPITER study, there was no low p-value: no reasonably certain difference in death rates comparing women either taking statins or not.[11] Oh, and the JUPITER trial was funded by AstraZeneca, the pharmaceutical company that makes the statin being tested in the study.

Statins forever?

It is now a couple of decades since I ate my cheesecake in coronary care. The patients whom I started on statins may still be taking them. Statins aren't like taking an antibiotic for a week to treat a chest infection, or even a few months' worth of an antidepressant.

When you are put on statins, the intention is that you will stay on them until you die.

Most trials of statins, however, take place over a few years. AFCAPS (Air Force/Texas Coronary Atherosclerosis Prevention Study) lasted just over five years. The PROSPER (The Prospective Study of Pravastatin in the Elderly at Risk) trial lasted just over three years. WOSCOPS, the West of Scotland Coronary Prevention Study, lasted almost five years. The Framingham data have been amassed over decades and continue to be collected. However, these are not statin RCTs but observational studies, where individuals are monitored and certain outcomes measured.

I'm rather keen to avoid harming my patients. When I sign off the prescriptions for statins, month after month, year after year, I'd like some data to reassure me. Are the drugs still necessary? Are they safe? Are there any problems relating to long-term prescriptions of statin medication?

We don't really know. Sure, there are ways to report side-effects of medicines to the government's agency – The Medicines and Healthcare Products Regulatory Agency (MHRA) – for ensuring medicines are reasonably safe, using the the internet or the traditional yellow postcards that doctors are supplied with for the purpose. But this method isn't failsafe. It may be hard to recognise a side-effect unless you look for it. Who would have guessed that diabetes was associated with statin use? In all honesty, the development of diabetes in someone on a statin – and who I therefore already knew to be at higher risk of vascular disease – wouldn't even make me blink twice, it would be so unexceptional. The best way to get reliable data about the side-effects of statins would be through actively looking for them in large studies.

Except there aren't many. Statins have been in regular use since the early 1990s. Few of the original trials have attempted follow-ups on the participants of primary prevention trials over longer periods. The follow-up to the WOSCOPS trial, for example, went back ten years later to find out what happened to the men in the west of Scotland who were part of the original trial. Researchers looked for all the typical things that statin trials do – heart attacks, strokes and all-cause mortality. Indeed they found a reduction in death rates, from 4.1% in the placebo group to 3.2% in the statin group. This just managed a 'significant' p-value, which was 0.051.[12]

While this tells us that in this study, there did seem to be a reduction in overall death rates, the chance of benefit was small. Five of the six authors of the paper reported receiving funding or some type of fee from the pharmaceutical industry.

There have been longer follow-ups from a few more statin trials but these have mainly been on patients who already have heart disease. One trial published in the *Lancet* in 2011 followed patients using statins for 11 years; however these were high-risk patients.[13] These groups of patients are important and do need to be studied but this still leaves a gap in knowledge, considering how much statin prescribing is now done in people at lower cardiovascular risk.

Sure, in some rare diseases it's pretty difficult to get long-term and reliable safety data about drugs and it may be that doctors and patients have to accept a large dollop of uncertainty when they are swallowing the medication. But here are millions of perfectly well people taking tablets with sparse trial data about long-term safety. It makes me uncomfortable. To paraphrase the famous quote of former US Defence Secretary Donald Rumsfeld, there are known knowns; there are things we know that we know. There are known unknowns. But there are also unknown unknowns – the things we don't know we don't know.

The Plain English Campaign gave Rumsfeld a 'Foot in Mouth' anti-award for his statement. Yet had he been talking about medical research, he would have been spot-on: we don't know what we don't know. We are blissful in our ignorance, unprepared to examine the things that aren't printed in medical journals. We assume that because we've done some measurements, we've calculated everything necessary.

That's why my pen often hovers hesitantly over a prescription. Are these statins really a good thing? But of course, it's not me taking them.

Blood pressure?

Whenever I read books about screening, even the few books that are critical about screening, blood pressure tends to skip gaily under the critical net. I have read media doctors who say that blood pressure (BP) should be checked at every opportunity, that cheap and widely available BP machines are as essential as paracetamol in the home medical kit. BP measuring is usually seen as good, even among those doctors and scientists who are more sceptical of screening.

May I dissent? We all have and need BP or we would be dead. When it's measured, you get two values, one above the other. The higher number refers to systolic pressure, and the lower number to the diastolic pressure. Low BP that is not caused by doctors (prescribing blood pressure treatments, usually) is rare, and manifests with dizziness, nausea and fainting. High BP, on the other hand, is roughly divided into two unequal types. One is 'malignant' hypertension, where a person has a very high BP (such as 200/140 or more) and signs of BP effects such as headache because of it. This small group have a disease and need urgent attention; they usually visit their doctor because they have symptoms of being unwell. The second, far larger, group, is of people with 'essential' hypertension. These people don't have symptoms of high BP, and they do not have a disease, but a risk marker for heart disease and stroke.

These are the people usually diagnosed via BP screenings. So what's normal? In 1989, if you were under 80 years old and your diastolic BP (the lower of the two BP reading numbers) was 100 or above, you merited medication. If your BP was just below that level, at between 95-99, then you were to be rechecked every few months.[14]

In 1993, treatment was extended to people with a diastolic BP over 90 if the person was over 60; younger patients with a diastolic BP between 90-99 were to be observed first.[15]

The third set of guidelines appeared in 1999. This introduced systolic pressure as a risk factor. Automatic treatment was to be started if your BP was over 160/100. If it was 140/90 and you had other signs of cardiovascular risk, you were to have your BP treated too.[16]

Now things became much more complicated. A BP of less than 135/85 was deemed normal, and even then, a recheck in five years was instructed. But at the next set of guidance, in 2004, 'normal' was no longer 135/85 but 130/85 ('high normal' was 130-139/85-89).[17] Seven years later, advisory body the National Institute for Health and Clinical Excellence (NICE) called 'stage 1 hypertension' a home monitoring average of 135/85 or over.[18]

We can see that over time, optimal BP has lowered. But how likely are we to postpone our death, or divert a heart attack or stroke, if we swallow the pills?

From Cochrane reviews, then: researchers found that, in order to prevent one cardiovascular 'event', 122 people with no prior heart attack or stroke had to be treated (the 'number needed to treat', or NNT) for 'mild' high BP – about 160mmHg systolic – with medication for five years.[19] That means a one in 122 chance of benefit; 121 times out of 122, you won't get a health advantage through taking the tablets. For people with moderate or severe high BP the potential for benefit of taking tablets was larger. They estimated that only 20 people had to be treated for five years to avoid one heart attack or stroke.

Is this impressive? 'Primary prevention' in treating high BP is common and thought of as the best in preventive drug interventions. Some types of patient may get more benefit from treatment than others. Cochrane reviews have also found, for example, that in African American women, treating high BP reduces all-cause mortality, with a NNT of 32 over five years.[20] Another Cochrane review concluded that you can reduce the risk of heart attack and stroke by treating hypertensive over-60s – but with provisos. The total mortality is what we want to know: there is no point avoiding death by stroke if the treatment makes you dizzy, you fall and fracture your hip, get pneumonia and die by that route instead. In the 60-80 age group, treatment could reduce deaths, but 84 people needed to be treated to delay one death. The over 80 group also had a reduction in heart attacks and strokes, but not in overall mortality rates.[21]

We are wedded to the idea that BP is bad and treatment is good. Elderly people think that they have a 40% risk of stroke without having their BP treated, and estimate that medication would halve their risk.[22] They are both over-optimistic and pessimistic: they don't have that high a risk of stroke, and the treatment for hypertension isn't that good.

My dissent is not that we should be against treating high BP. My argument is against unthinking treatment of high BP. Taking medication for it probably won't save your life so if the tablets make you feel miserable, your doctor and you need to take an honest look at the evidence and your priorities.

To the church hall

To my NHS and my home address, I've had letters inviting me to come to have cardiovascular screening. The company that offers this, Life Line Screening, tends to set itself up in church halls after drumming up local interest with a leafleting campaign in the area. The letter starts:

> 'Did you know that cardiovascular disease is the number one killer of men <u>and</u> women in the UK – and a leading cause of permanent disability? Unfortunately, <u>many significant cardiovascular problems lie dormant and show no symptoms</u> until there are potentially serious complications.'

They also say: 'Many of our customers have an annual screening as part of their regular healthcare regime'. 'Customer' is a word slipped in just the same at most of the other screening clinics. The word 'patient' has disappeared, swallowed up by the modern mantra of choice, feeding the notion that 'customers' are empowered beings with credit cards, exerting their right to choose what they want.

Yet what we know of addressing vascular risk is complex, and there is no clear path for us to tread. When doctors learn, train and practise the art of professionalism, they are taught the ethical practices of medicine. The very core is this: doctors are powerful because of the knowledge they have and the trust that most people give to them. Doctors must not abuse this. Doctors must treat patients with honesty, must not take advantage, and must use evidence to guide their approach.

The regulatory body for doctors, the General Medical Council, says: 'In providing care you must . . . provide effective treatments based on the best possible evidence.'[23] When you replace the doctor-patient relationship with a doctor-customer relationship, there is almost no point in having a doctor in the equation. Customers are entitled to ask and pay for whatever they wish, no matter how ludicrous, dangerous, unnecessary or unhelpful the order is.

A patient, treated by a doctor with professionalism, should be supplied with unbiased information, which is not pitched at filling a purse. A patient should be given evidence serving to control the excesses of medicine being thrown wildly at her. A patient should be given the benefit of medical knowledge and experience in a way that enables doctor and patient to be on the same side, helping each other make good decisions – not sexing up and selling tests for the sake of a business deal.

3

The nature of cancer:
breast beating

Bizarre, but true: if we cut out screening for cancer, we'd reduce the amount of cancer we diagnose. But surely, you say, this would just mean that we would diagnose life-threatening illnesses 'too late'? Wouldn't this stop us getting better treatment earlier? We'd get more cancer deaths, wouldn't we?

Not necessarily. Once again, the facts are complex and counterintuitive.

Cancer is not always a very bad thing. Cancer can painlessly co-exist with a person, not causing any symptoms, not causing any trouble. We have become accustomed to reflexively equating cancer with a death sentence. We think of cancer and we think of surgery, chemotherapy and the need for a will.

This isn't an accurate reflection of what cancer is. The word describes a vast amount of tissue changes, ranging from the indolent and lazy to the genuinely life shortening and difficult to treat. The truth is that many people harbour cancers that we know nothing about, and they die of something else.

We know this because pathologists often find unexpected cancers during postmortem examination, where the cancer had nothing to do with the patient's death. For example, a study published in the *Journal of the American Medical Association* (*JAMA*) in 1987 looked at postmortem lung cancer diagnoses over almost ten years. Out of the 2,996 postmortem examinations carried out, 110 showed lung cancer that had already been suspected. But in 26 other patients, a diagnosis of lung cancer was made out of the blue; what the researchers termed a 'surprise'.[1] Another study using postmortem examinations looked at unsuspected cancer rates in the US. It found that 7% of the examinations done discovered a cancer that had been unsuspected – and which was nothing to do with the patient's death.[2] In the journal *Human Pathology*, in 1994, Swedish pathologists described how, in a series of just over 3,000 postmortems, around one in 20 people had an undiagnosed and unsuspected cancer.[3] It's clear from this research that we can have cancer in our bodies that we don't suspect and that will not kill or harm us. We shall die having had no symptoms from this cancer, and from a cause unrelated to it. We have to factor this in when we think about screening healthy people for disease.

DCIS – a hidden disease?

Take ductal carcinoma in situ (DCIS). This is a breast condition that hardly existed before breast screening started. If you ask a doctor what breast cancer looks like, chances are they will describe a lump either on the breast or within the axilla, or breast skin that looks tethered or pulled. DCIS isn't any of these things, It's a condition that is seen on X-ray, or mammogram, as fine, granular changes. The DCIS cells are confined to the milk duct of the breast rather than extending outside it, meaning that it is contained ('in situ'). Radiologists use magnifying glasses or enlarged digital images to help identify minute patterns that may point to a potential problem.

DCIS makes up a large chunk of breast cancer diagnoses given at screening: 28.2% of breast cancer diagnosed in US women aged 40-49 at screening is DCIS, falling to 16% in women aged 70-84.[4] A common treatment for DCIS is to remove the entire breast; 30% of women with DCIS have removal of the breast – mastectomy.[5] How much of this treatment is necessary?

What is known is that only a minority of DCIS goes on to become a life-threatening cancer and even that knowledge is built on wobbly foundations. The most reliable evidence of what happens to DCIS over time is based on just 28 women who had biopsy-proven DCIS but did not have any further surgical removal of the area. These women have now been followed up for an average of 30 years. Seven developed invasive breast cancer within ten years. One further invasive cancer was diagnosed 15 years after the initial biopsy, and three others between 23 and 42 years afterwards. Five of these 28 women died of breast cancer. Seventeen of the 28 did not go on to develop invasive breast cancer.[6]

So what exactly is DCIS? Is it cancer, a pre-cancer, or what? The honest answer is that despite providing breast screening tests every three years to British women between the ages of 50 and 64, and on request thereafter, and diagnosing DCIS thousands of times per year, we are not terribly sure.

We are certainly diagnosing it more often when we perform breast screening. A systematic review of the published evidence in the *Journal of the National Cancer Institute* in the US, published in 2009, found that the rate of DCIS diagnosis had increased from 1.87 per 100,000 women in the early 1970s to 32.5 per 100,000 women in 2004.[7] It is now also known that many women die with DCIS, rather than from it. From studies of autopsies published in the *Annals of Internal Medicine*, 1.3% of women were found to have invasive breast cancer and 8.9% had DCIS. None of these women were known to have breast cancer during their lives.[8] The actual rate of DCIS might be higher because some pathologists may not routinely search hard for a finding of no significance to the cause of death. So, DCIS is increasing in rate of diagnosis; it is found more when we perform breast screening. It does not often behave as an aggressive cancer but is treated as one, often with mastectomy.

Diagnosing cancers that were never going to cause harm incurs the risk of overtreating women. A minority of DCIS will progress to invasive cancers, but no one can be sure which ones. This means that more women are treated with mastectomy than will benefit from it.

Mastectomy is a major operation, often requiring reconstruction either at the time or later. It requires general anaesthetic, and complications include infection, bleeding and scarring. It causes disruption and distress personally, to family and to work life, and affects other issues such as medical insurance. A steady climb in the amount of DCIS diagnosed has led to an increasing number of mastectomies, with the amount doubling to more than 900 operations a year in the UK between 1998 and 2008. As one breast surgeon put it:

> 'DCIS has an excellent long-term outlook and there are concerns that many patients with DCIS would not have developed an invasive cancer if left untreated. The issue in relation to DCIS therefore has to be avoiding potential overtreatment because few women die as a consequence of having DCIS . . .'[9]

If breast surgeons think that they are operating too often for DCIS, what about the view of a woman diagnosed with DCIS, writing about her treatment?

> '. . . the reality of this diagnosis has been two wide excisions, one partial mutilation (sorry, mastectomy), one reconstruction, five weeks' radiotherapy (a 60-mile round trip and I had to pay to park), chronic infection at the donor site, one nipple reconstruction, seven general anaesthetics, and more than a year off work . . . I expect that I have been classified as a screening success. Yet, everything about my experience tells me the opposite. Screening has caused me considerable and lasting harm. It has certainly not saved or prolonged my life, which is the purpose of screening.'[10]

Even the most fervent breast screening supporter should admit that screening may have nasty flipsides. Jane Flanders, the woman who wrote that searing letter to the *BMJ*, may well have had an indolent DCIS that would have had no impact on her life. Surely anyone who cared about women and their autonomy would want the uncertainties and risks of breast screening shared with the very women who were being asked to undergo the testing and subsequent interventions? Wouldn't they? Not on your life.

In 2004 I was asked to speak at a meeting organised by the charity Breast Cancer Care, in Westminster. The subject was 'The screening age range and the interval and information given to patients about screening'. The meeting was chaired by former Conservative MP Edwina Currie, who lost no time in proudly describing her role as the health minister responsible for setting up the NHS Breast Screening Programme in 1988 after her government came into power having pledged to introduce it during campaigning in the previous year.[11]

During the debate it became clear that DCIS was not on the radar of most screening enthusiasts. Afterwards, I asked Currie what she thought of the information women were given about the problems with a DCIS diagnosis before they had the screening test. Her answer? It shocked me so much that I wrote it down in my diary immediately afterwards: 'I've never heard of it.' She appeared quite unembarrassed. Her answer is not surprising, given that she is also on record as saying: 'In political terms, with the elections no more than a few months away (breast screening) was also attractive.'[12]

Was the whole breast screening programme less about science and more about being a pink-ribboned vote winner?

Does breast screening work?

This big question goes beyond DCIS. Over the past decade there has been the occasional public surfacing of spats involving breast screeners versus the more determinedly evidence-based and sceptical doctors, researchers and patients. Despite a general acknowledgment of the limitations and problems with screening in the medical community – disagreements about the level of benefit cause far more angst – there has been little practical movement towards telling the people who might just want to know – the women themselves.

So what do we know?

If you rely on the NHS Breast Screening Programme for

advice, you will be told, in its most recent leaflet published in December 2010, that:

'Regular screening prevents deaths from breast cancer.

Screening can find cancer early, before you know it's there. The earlier breast cancer is found, the better your chance of surviving it.

If a breast cancer is found early, you are less likely to have a mastectomy (your breast removed) or chemotherapy.'

It goes on:

'What are the downsides of being screened?

Having a mammogram means your breasts are exposed to a small amount of radiation.

Sometimes a mammogram will look normal, even if a cancer is there. This is called a false negative result. You should remain *breast aware*.

Sometimes a mammogram will not look normal and you will be recalled for further tests, but cancer is not there. This is called a false positive result.

Screening can find cancers which are treated but which may not otherwise have been found during your lifetime.

If you go for screening you may be anxious or worried. This usually only lasts for a short time.'

The statistics the programme quotes read:

'The numbers are current *best estimates* but may change over time.

Breast cancer is the most common cancer in women. There are around 46,000 cases a year in the UK. Eight out of ten breast cancers are found in women aged 50 and over.

About 12,000 women die of breast cancer each year in the UK.

For every 14,000 women screened regularly for ten years, one woman may develop breast cancer she will die from because of radiation from the mammograms.

About 8 out of every 1,000 women screened will be found to

have breast cancer. Of these, two will be told they have an early form of cancer called ductal carcinoma in situ (DCIS). We don't know which cases of DCIS will become harmful so we offer these women treatment . . .

For every 400 women screened regularly for ten years, one less will die from breast cancer. This means that around 1,400 women are prevented from dying from breast cancer each year in England.'[13]

This makes a fairly definite case for breast cancer screening. The message is that breast screening saves lives, and could save yours.

But are these statistical estimates fair? How many people have to have breast screening in order to prevent one death from breast cancer? The NHS is telling us that they have to screen 400 women to stop one death from breast cancer.

Where does this number come from? Here it gets interesting. The numbers quoted were cited four years before the leaflet was published, in an 'executive summary', written by the Advisory Committee on Breast Cancer Screening, and printed in the *Journal of Medical Screening*. The abstract from this journal says:

'For every 400 women screened regularly by the NHSBSP over a ten year period, one woman fewer will die from breast cancer than would have died without screening.'[14]

However there was no individual reference given to support this statement, other than to say that there was 'an extensive body of research'.

The Committee's full report was published by the NHS.[15] This time, the statistics were backed up with the comment that the debate on the effectiveness of screening 'had been largely resolved in 2002 by a report from the international working group of the IARC', the International Agency for Research on Cancer. This 'expert working group' met in Lyon in France to discuss the current state of affairs in the breast screening world back in 2002.

When they met, the situation was slightly odd. They were experts in their field being asked to look at the published research in the area. Their conclusions would be important – indeed, the numbers they found are still being quoted by the NHS in 2011.

The agency's published report takes the form of an examination of research and then an assessment, with detailed comments on the various randomised controlled trials that have been done of screening mammograms. These are difficult studies to interpret if you are trying to decide if breast screening is a good thing. Treatments for breast cancer have improved enormously over the past few decades, with different chemotherapy and hormone-based therapies being used to target and kill cancer cells. If you find studies saying that screening saves lives, how can you be sure it is the screening, and not better treatment causing the positive effect? Perhaps it doesn't matter if the cancer is diagnosed a bit sooner by screening or detected by the woman herself if the treatment is of high quality.

There is another problem. If it looks like breast cancer screening is picking up more cancers, this is likely to include a lot of DCIS. But while DCIS is frequently diagnosed at screening, as we have seen, its progress is less certain. It does not always kill or even maim. Your numbers will indicate successful treatment, but most of those lives were never under threat.

The report is detailed and clearly intent on trying to establish if screening works or not. The difficulty with it is that it has been written by a committee trying to reach a consensus. Much of the data are based on estimate and approximation.

The report concludes, in a chapter on effectiveness, that:

'The effect of screening is real but small at present, the estimates of change in national overall breast cancer mortality rates being 5-10% in countries with the longest experience. The estimates were larger in a few studies of sub-populations and after removal of bias due to deaths in cases diagnosed before the start of screening . . . The gain in life years per screen is nevertheless likely to remain small . . . Although screening for breast cancer may thus appear to be insufficiently effective for use as public health policy, that conclusion is probably not justified. Screening for breast cancer also has a humanitarian value, in addition to the prolongation of life. Screening, in principle, offers a greater chance to select the type of intervention, including breast conserving and less invasive treatment. Most recalls are due to false-positive results, which cause unnecessary anxiety and invasive or otherwise unpleasant investigations. A decision on whether to screen should depend on a weighing of all the effects and how they compare with other health services . . . '[16]

This doesn't exactly read like a paean to screening. It sounds far more like a high-wire balancing act, where the potential for good sways above deep and troubling uncertainties. It also runs against the more recent studies, previously discussed, which have noted that more screening leads to more mastectomy. As for false positive results, we can include much DCIS in this tally, which means that 'unpleasant treatment' can include mastectomy – with, potentially, complications like those described by Jane Flanders in the *BMJ*.

What happens when you take the experts out and just look at the evidence? Experts can be a source of bias simply because they are experts: if a study came out saying that your own specialty, your entire research and life's work, was a waste of time, it might not be easy to accept. Doctors tend to be vocational people who want to do good things: if you found out that your 'good thing' was to cause the deaths of thousands of babies or cancer in millions of smokers you might react, at least initially, with a measure of disbelief. We all have vested interests.

A famous story: cardiologists were suspicious when Archie Cochrane wanted to study their units to find out if longer inpatient stays harmed patients. He did the work and showed them the results: longer cardiology stays were good for patients. The pleased cardiologists agreed the data proved their units worked. Then Cochrane told them that he had actually reversed the numbers. They had to accept the unthinkable; longer stays harmed patients.*

---

* I have tried my best to mitigate and reduce my own bias by having an attractive back-up plan should general practice be proven to be a dangerous sham. I will switch seamlessly to writing children's stories, organising children's science parties and providing buffet catering for a living.

There are a few people who have denounced the push to breast screening, and I regard them as heroes of our time. These include the surgeon Michael Baum, who was involved in setting up breast cancer screening before calling attention to its potential harms. Peter Gøtzsche, Margrethe Nielsen and Karsten Jørgensen work from the Nordic Cochrane Centre in Denmark. They have persistently completed Cochrane reviews of the literature around breast screening, publishing their findings and answering to their detractors. They identified eleven relevant trials about breast screening, excluding two because they were not designed to answer the question of whether or not breast screening reduced mortality or morbidity. They assessed each trial for bias; for example, one trial run in Edinburgh was biased because 26% of the control group were from higher social classes compared with 56% of the study group. Because social class is related to breast cancer risk, these unbalanced groups couldn't be fairly compared. This means that the study wasn't reliable and it therefore wasn't included in the overall assessment. The review concludes:

'Despite the shortcomings of the trials, screening appears to lower breast cancer mortality. However, the chance that a woman will benefit from attending screening is very small, and considerably smaller than the risk that she may experience harm. It is thus not clear whether screening does more good than harm. Women, clinicians and policy makers should consider the trade-offs carefully when they decide whether or not to attend or support screening programs.'[17]

Their findings about the benefits and harms of breast screening do not reflect what women in the UK are told when they are 'invited' to screening (at an appointment that has been been pre-arranged). Based on their research, they have published an alternative breast cancer screening information leaflet, which is freely available on their website:

'It may be reasonable to attend for breast cancer screening with mammography, but it may also be reasonable not to attend because screening has both benefits and harms.

If 2,000 women are screened regularly for ten years, one will benefit from the screening, as she will avoid dying from breast cancer.

At the same time, 10 healthy women will, as a consequence, become cancer patients and will be treated unnecessarily. These women will have either a part of their breast or the whole breast removed, and they will often receive radiotherapy and sometimes chemotherapy.

Furthermore, about 200 healthy women will experience a false alarm. The psychological strain until one knows whether it was cancer, and even afterwards, can be severe.'[18]

Talking of harm

There are uncertainties over whether cases of DCIS will develop into invasive cancer. We also know that the radiation from X-rays in screening mammograms causes a few new breast cancers. The NHS estimates (and it is an estimate, no one knows for sure) that for every 14,000 women being screened in the UK over ten years (which means one screening every three years within that timespan), there is 'about' one fatal breast cancer due to the screening.[19] A 2010 paper in the US journal *Radiology* worked out that for every 100,000 women, screened annually between the ages of 40 to 55 and then every second year to age of 74, there would be 86 cancers and 11 deaths caused by the radiation. Those doctors concluded that 'The risk of radiation-induced breast cancer should not be a deterrent from mammographic screening'[20] but they miss the point. *They* think it shouldn't be a deterrent to screening. But why not let the women who are going for screening decide for themselves?

It simply isn't fair for these individuals to make a value judgment for you, no matter how good their intentions. That's the thing about value – you have to decide what yours are. Our values are personal; they don't belong to someone else.

Rumsfeld was right. You also have to think about the unknown unknowns. The harms you don't yet know.

If something untoward shows on the mammogram, you need some tissue to put under a microscope to help decide what it is. Breast biopsy is part of 'triple assessment' – examination, mammogram and biopsy – used in order to delineate a breast lump.

We already know about the harm caused by anxiety and false positives and unnecessary mastectomies – but could the biopsy itself also cause harm?

Possibly but again, we don't really know. A literature review performed in 2010 concluded that: 'There is histological evidence of seeding of tumour cells from the primary neoplastic site into adjacent breast tissue, following biopsy.' In other words, the action of inserting a needle into the area of concern could spread cancer cells into the surrounding area.[21]

Now, this hasn't been shown to spread cancer in a life-endangering way. But it is yet another question mark hovering somewhere in the equation asking: 'Is breast screening doing more harm than good? Does it lead us to take actions whereby we may create more problems than we solve?'

The 'unknown unknowns' are vast. It may even be impossible to think about and address every one of them. But when we are inviting perfectly well patients to have screening tests intending to improve their health, we need to know we aren't harming them more. The facts are quite different from the pink-tinted messages women get about breast screening.

4

Smears and fears:
the Jade Goody effect

Cervical screening has been running in the UK since 1964. When Jade Goody, a television celebrity, died of cervical cancer in 2009, there was a rise in the number of women attending for smear tests, with the future prime minister, David Cameron, saying: 'Her legacy will be to save the lives of more young women in the future.'[1] More screening was simply a good thing.

Cervical screening – the smear test – should have several of the qualities of an ideal screening test. The cells in the cervix – the tissue at the top of the vagina, the 'neck' of the womb – can become cancerous, almost always in response to HPV, a sexually transmitted virus that is a member of the 'cold sore' virus family. However, after infection, cervical cancer – should it develop – usually takes years to occur. During this time, 'pre-cancerous' cells can form. The hope with cervical screening is that by taking a sample of these cells from the cervix of women who have no symptoms, very early cellular changes can be identified and removed, or treated with heat or laser.

In the waiting room at my workplace, there are large pink posters, fronted by smiling attractive women, asking you to 'Make time for your smear test'. Cancer Research UK produced some leaflets saying that 'most cases of cervical cancer could be prevented' and 'What affects your risk?' Top of the list: 'If you don't go for screening doctors will not be able to find and treat any early changes in your cervix. These changes could then lead to cervical cancer.'[2] The NHS says 'Put it on your list' and even manages to put 'go for screening test' in between 'book haircut' and 'buy cinema tickets.'[3]

In the face of such pointed and well-meaning pressure, dissent would seem churlish at best. Not pitching up for your smear would seem as daft as crossing the road with your eyes closed.

But is it? What we actually know about cervical screening is far from clear — making it slightly more complex than choosing what colour highlights to have.

Angela Raffle, a public health doctor in Bristol, has produced some of the most illuminating research about how effective the cervical smear test is. She and her colleagues published a paper in the *BMJ* in 2003, which analysed the effect of cervical screening amongst the 350,000 women in the Bristol area she worked in and organised cervical screening for. The results are disturbing because they rub against the straightforward logic about screening presented to us by its proponents. I quote:

> 'For every 10,000 women screened from 1976 to 1996, 1,564 had abnormal cytology,* 818 were investigated, and 543 had abnormal histology.** 176 had persistent abnormality for two years or more. In the absence of screening, 80 women would be expected to develop cancer of the cervix by 2011, of whom 25 would die.
>
> With screening ten of these deaths could be avoided. . . . The lifetime risk for having abnormal cytology detected could be as high as 40% for women born since 1960.'[4]

Let's recap. Without screening, over 20 years, 25 out of 10,000 women would die. With screening, taking the same group over the same period of time, 15 would die of cervical cancer. Only ten – the difference between 25 and 15 – out of the 10,000 benefited

---

    *   cell changes detected at cervical smear
   **   cell changes detected after examination of a cervical biopsy, done at colposcopy

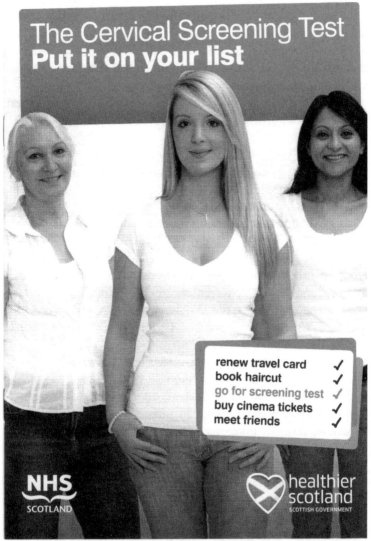

Haircuts and smear tests: the cover of NHS Scotland's cervical screening test leaflet

from screening by having their lives extended.

Ten women out of every 10,000 over 20 years isn't, of course, an unimportant number. But it's not the only number here. To stop these deaths from cervical cancer, you have to do a lot more tests on a lot more women. A total of 818 women had invasive tests, namely biopsy. A biopsy can be taken using an adapted microscope, which examines the cervix, and can treat areas of abnormal cells, in a process called colposcopy. Of these biopsies, 543 had an abnormal result. Two had cancer, 22 had 'micro-invasive' cancer, 361 had high-grade dysplasia, and 158 had low-grade abnormalities.

Isn't all this worth it? After all, as we are told by the NHS, it could save your life. Perhaps, perhaps not. 'Anxiety' is often mentioned as a 'minor' side-effect of screening. It's said so lightly as though it hardly matters. But anxiety as a side-effect does matter. Some women are made ill from worry when a letter arrives on their doorstep telling them that their smear is abnormal and that they need further tests. Women can become sleepless, imagining infertility, early death and their children growing up without a mother. Some women manage to put this to one side and get on with their other concerns; some don't. It can be a pervasive worry and a recurrent fear. Anxiety isn't just a minor side-effect.

Colposcopy may just involve inspection of the female genitals. It may also involve treatment to the cervix. In the UK, a common treatment is 'large loop excision of the transformation zone' (LLETZ) where the abnormal cells are removed under local anaesthetic. It's popular because it's quick, can be done immediately and doesn't need an overnight stay in hospital. But it is associated with problems later – namely preterm birth. Women who have had this procedure are more likely to have a baby born before full term.[5] One Canadian study found that 2.5% of women who hadn't had a LLETZ procedure gave birth prematurely, as opposed to 7.9% who had.[6]

Is it worth the risk? It might be. It depends on your perspective. A woman may feel that a small chance of stopping a death from cervical cancer is worth the downsides, such as LLETZ procedures that do not benefit the patient and raise the risk of premature birth. Or she may not. What if she had several anxiety-inducing smears, biopsies, and treatment with no benefit to her?

I can't answer that question. But I do feel deep discomfort that these issues aren't raised with women routinely before having a smear test. The government may have decided that the smear test is a good thing; but that may not correspond to the woman's own wishes.

With cervical screening, Angela Raffle's study says the potential good is a reduction in cervical cancer deaths from 25 to 15, per 10,000 women, per 20 years. The cost of achieving this means that almost 1,000 other women get letters telling them they have abnormalities and need repeat tests. More than 500 require colposcopy and biopsy, with the risk that this may lead to premature labour in later pregnancies.

Despite the easy lure of government posters, cervical screening is not a simple experience akin to a visit to the cinema. It isn't a clear cut situation of good versus bad, but a balancing of potential gains and harms. Doctors should not assume that you want to make this trade. Doctors should help you decide what you want to do; explain the risks, not just decide that you value the chance of gain enough to accept the potential of harm.

Personally, I think that the overselling and oversimplification of this difficult melange of pros and cons we currently have is a patronising outrage. It's oversexed health advice; overselling of a complex test with many outcomes, not all good. The losers are us, the 'customers', who are simply enticed into screening.

The real story of cervical screening

Cervical cancer is relatively rare. Only two out of every 100 cancers diagnosed in women are cervical. The female population of the UK is 30.2 million strong, and the most recent figures available show that around 2,800 women are diagnosed with cervical cancer every year.[7]

The Cancer Research Campaign website shows a nice, pink-lined graph of the death rate from cervical cancer falling over the past 30 years. In 1971, eight women per 100,000 died of cervical cancer; now the rate is around two per 100,000.

Many people – notably those working in cervical screening – would like to attribute this to screening. They point to the fact that, after cervical screening started, death rates fell. But dig back further. Look back another couple of decades. It is the National Statistics Authority that notes:

'From 1950 to 1987 . . . mortality from cervical cancer in England and Wales fell steadily from just over 1.5 per cent every year from 11.2 per 100,000 to 6.1 per 100,000. This long term decline in cervical cancer mortality predates the introduction of screening, and may be due to improvements in hygiene and nutrition, the shifting of childbearing patterns towards smaller family sizes, delayed childbearing and increased mean age at first birth; and a decline in sexually transmitted diseases.'[8]

In other words, deaths from cervical cancer were falling before screening started. So can we be sure that screening is causing the reduced death rates?

If you wanted to find out whether or not cervical screening reduced deaths from cervical cancer, you'd want to do a trial – a trial fairly comparing what happens when you screen women for cervical cancer versus not screening them. (Remember, this is not about looking after women with symptoms that could mean cervical cancer – only women who were well and who had no symptoms.) Knowing that other factors were reducing deaths from cervical cancer, you'd want to be sure that it was screening

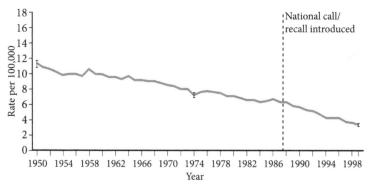

Death rates from cervical cancer: the last 60 years.[8]

– not something else, like a reduction in child-bearing – that was making the improvement. So you would set up a trial with two groups, identical but for one thing – cervical smears – monitor them and see what happened.

So, do we have this kind of trial evidence? Nope. The American Society for the Control of Cancer (now the American Cancer Society) was set up in 1913 with the express aim of showing the world that cancer could be cured if caught early. In the 1940s, a New York researcher, Dr George Papanicolaou, developed a cell-staining technique that he said could identify abnormal cervical cells taken from vaginal fluid.[9] Momentum gathered. The *JAMA* reported, in 1961, Dr Curtis Lund's address to its annual meeting – An Epitaph for Cervical Carcinoma – in which he said that the 'means for eliminating cervical carcinoma as a cause of death are now available' through pelvic examination (internal vaginal physical examination), cervical smears to all women over twenty – and women under twenty who had ever been pregnant – together with biopsies and 'appropriate surgical therapy.'[10] He spoke to influential medics and a world afraid of the 'Big C'. Yet, when these North American doctors started to use smear tests and evangelically took the test to the world's women, 'definitive data that it saved lives hardly existed at this time.'[11]

In 1979, the *Lancet* published a paper that attempted to examine the impact that cervical smears had made in women who had developed cervical cancer. The researchers looked back to see how often women with cervical cancer had smears compared to a matched group of women without cervical cancer. The result seemed to support screening. Women with cervical cancer were less likely to have had a smear.

But does this prove that cervical screening saved lives? No. There are other reasons that could explain the difference. For example, women at highest risk for cervical cancer – women who had multiple sexual partners or who smoked – may have wished to avoid doctors and not attend for smears. The most health-conscious and least risk-taking women may have been more likely to attend for smears. It may have been these attitudes towards risk that protected the women, rather than the smear tests. If you want to work out what smear tests do with a higher and more reliable degree of certainty, the best way is still through a randomised controlled trial; a fair test, where we try to reduce the play of chance to a minimum and find out whether smears could make a difference.

The authors of that 1979 *Lancet* paper realised this but didn't think a high-quality trial was going to be possible. They wrote:

'There is still some uncertainty about the efficiency of the screening programme which uses the Papanicolaou (Pap) smear in reducing the incidence of invasive cervical cancer. This uncertainty will probably persist until a properly randomised controlled trial has been carried out, but unfortunately such a trial is impractical. Several non-randomised studies have given encouraging results, but such studies are liable to self-selection bias [when the women with lowest risks for cancer attend for screening most regularly], with the screened women tending to be of higher socioeconomic status than the unscreened and thus less likely to get cervical cancer.'[12]

Why did they think that such a trial was impractical? They cited a paper in the journal *Cancer*, co-written in 1977 by a doctor, Maureen Henderson, and a professor from the Department of Social and Preventive Medicine at the University of Maryland, which stated that:

'Given the unacceptability of conducting a rigorous randomised controlled trial of an ongoing and accepted cancer control procedure, an alternative experimental approach is proposed.'[13]

What they wanted to do was compare 'normally' screened women to screened women who were vigorously tracked down and encouraged to come in for tests. Yet this still would not have proved definitively whether the cervical screening test worked or not. What seems extraordinary is that these doctors felt that there was doubt about how useful cervical screening was, yet did not feel that they could recommend high-quality trials to establish firmly what was going on. For example, they go on to say:

'It is difficult if not impossible to estimate from this analysis of available vital statistics how much of the fall in invasive cervical cancer death rates is the result of continued improvement in general hygiene and medical care and how much is the direct result of disease control programs based on early detection with exfoliative cytology [cervical screening]'.

They add:

'Randomised controlled clinical trials . . . have recently been viewed as the ultimate method for the acquisition of evaluative information. They are, however, cumbersome research tools which face ethical constraints when used to evaluate established health programs.'[13]

The irony is astounding. The real ethical issue was subjecting millions of women to a program that hadn't been tested to a high standard. Instead of declaring that better data were desperately needed, they were effectively saying that it was impossible to challenge the status quo. In doing so, they condemned future generations to unnecessary uncertainty over whether cervical cancer deaths were being reduced by screening.

What do we know now? We still don't have high-quality randomised controlled trials to guide our decisions. Many prominent statisticians are firmly of the view that cervical screening saves lives. For example, Professor Sir Julian Peto wrote in the *Lancet* in 2004 that:

'Cervical screening has prevented an epidemic that would have killed about one in 65 of all British women born since 1950 and culminated in about 6,000 deaths per year in this country. However, these estimates are subject to substantial uncertainty, particularly in relation to the effects of oral contraceptives and changes in sexual behaviour. 80% or more of these deaths (up to 5,000 deaths per year) are likely to be prevented by screening . . .'[14]

'Substantial uncertainty'? I'll say. To reach this conclusion, which was reported in the media with great enthusiasm, Peto and his colleagues analysed international trends in mortality rates from cervical cancer, before and after screening was introduced. He had no control group, unlike a clinical trial which would be able to compare the effect of the smear in one group with the effect of having no smear in another. Peto and his colleagues instead examined the deaths from cervical cancer in groups of women of different ages. He found that as time went on there were fewer deaths from cervical cancer. He extrapolated this forwards and concluded that criticisms of the programme were unjustified. But the conclusions were based on analysing trends and are therefore subject to more uncertainty than a trial would be.

But never mind. Here is the director of the NHS Cancer Screening Programme welcoming Peto's results:

'I am delighted that these findings recognise the huge contribution that the cervical screening programme has made to saving women's lives. We work hard to set the highest standards to ensure that women can access our world leading, high quality cervical screening programme. As this research shows, regular screening is one of the best defences against cervical cancer and so I urge all women to attend when invited.'[15]

Indeed, women are urged to get a smear test, and not to ask questions or clarify any doubts they might have about the uncertainty or risk involved. Any operation on the human body needs 'informed consent', when doctors must be honest about the chances of harm as well as benefit. Why is it any different for screening? We still lack high-quality research data about the impact of cervical screening on death rates. Women have a much higher chance of a false positive test than of having their life prolonged by it. Yet we are coy about the harms and the problems of screening: why?

Part of the problem is that doctors, who should have been shouting loud and long for proper scientific method and proof amid the clamour for smear tests, have stayed quiet. A rare few spoke out, such as Archie Cochrane who, when head of the epidemiology unit at the Medical Research Council in the early

70s, said 'never has there been less appeal to evidence and more to opinion' than when cervical screening was discussed.[11] He was branded a heretic by other doctors. What were we afraid of?

More isn't more

When Jade Goody died *The Sun* newspaper, best known for pictures of topless women, ran a campaign to lower the age for cervical screening from 25 to 20. The cervical screening programme had previously invited women between the ages of 20-25 but after a change in policy in 2003, this was changed so that the first smear was done at age 25.[16] Goody's death spurred a movement to screen women earlier, and fury that under 25s were not being currently included in the programme boiled from the press. One 23-year-old wrote indignantly in *The Guardian*:

> 'I recently visited my GP and asked for a smear. I was refused because of my age. There was no proper explanation, and like most people I followed doctor's orders. But then I started to think that, as cervical cancer is symptomless at first, I could have it, but I won't know for another two years or until it shows symptoms. I'm not alone in feeling frustrated – many women under 25, encouraged by Jade Goody's very public discussion of her cancer, are using social networking sites to discuss being refused smears . . . refusing women smear tests is infuriatingly counterintuitive.'[17]

This illustrates the extent to which cervical screening has become a protective talisman. For that 23-year-old, there is no good evidence that screening would do her any good; and much more evidence that it could do her harm. In young women, 'abnormal' changes are so frequent that they are not a good guide to the likelihood of cervical cancer developing later. Nevertheless, numerous health charities joined in the mêlée. For example, sexual healthcare charity Marie Stopes International issued a press release saying:

'Cervical cancer, while extremely rare among women under 30, does nevertheless represent a potential threat to their lives and wellbeing . . . an about-turn from the Government to offer screening from a younger age could save lives.'[18]

To that end, an extraordinary meeting of the governmental Advisory Committee on Cervical Screening was convened. The committee noted that when the minimum screening age had been changed from 20 to 25 in 2004, there had been no change in the number of cases of cervical cancer in that age group. Yet it is minuted that Mr Robert Music, director of cancer charity Jo's Trust, said that 'screening did not cause harm' and that 'there was enormous public support for the age to be reduced, with over 200,000 signatures on recent petitions.'[19]

The idea that cervical screening doesn't do any harm is nonsense. For women under 25, 29% will have an abnormal smear – their cervix is prone to giving false positives, where the cells look 'abnormal' but are actually normal for that age group.[20] In a study of 1,781 women with 'mild' dyskaryosis (mild cervical cell changes), examined between 1965 and 1984, invasive cancers later occurred in ten women at long-term follow-up, and 46% of abnormal smears returned to normal appearances with no treatment and within two years.[21]

Clearly, having an abnormal smear is common, but having cervical cancer is not common. How do you know which abnormal smears are the risky ones? No one knows, and so all women with abnormal smears are followed up, with more smears and more colposcopy, with all the complications that entails: pain, bleeding, infection, worry, anxiety and, rarely, sustained bleeding that requires pressure packs and catheters. A smear test is certainly not a simple, benign procedure; it can lead to unanticipated consequences.

But isn't it worth it if it saves lives? That would depend on there being any evidence that lives were saved (or deaths delayed) in the under-25 age group at all. The *BMJ* published a study in 2009 examining age groups in relation to the effectiveness of cervical cancer screening. This was a case control study, not quite as good as a randomised controlled trial, but based on real life

Case control study

A group of patients with condition X are identified. This group is the matched with another group of patients, aiming to be identical but for the presence of the disease.

The groups are compared with each other, looking for factors which could help to explain differences in rates of condition X.

A major problem with this type of study is recall bias, for example, remembering reliably what kind of food or how much alcohol was consumed in the past. Another problem can be the difficulty in creating fairly, otherwise identically matched groups.

data and able to compare what happened in different groups of women having smears. Just over 4,000 women diagnosed with invasive cervical cancer were matched with women who did not have cancer, and differences between the groups were looked at. They found no evidence at all that screening women aged under 25 reduced cervical cancer incidence.[22] If we were more critical, we could say that all we offered to under-25s was invasive and possibly harmful procedures.

Over 18 years, the authors found 73 women diagnosed with cervical cancer and who were between the ages of 20 and 24. Only five of them had *not* been screened previously – this was not a group of women who didn't bother with screening tests.

The obvious conclusion is that cervical screening is not very effective at stopping these young women from developing cervical cancer. But what did the advisory committee do? Did it reflect the evidence and inform women that they were only being damaged, not helped, by starting smear tests earlier? No: the committee proposed a 'fig leaf' of sending out invitations for screening to women aged 24 and a half.

Screening: misunderstood, and misunderstood again

Even more concerning in the minutes of the advisory committee's meeting is the muddle over what screening actually means. One woman, a representative from a health charity, says:

> 'I've spoken to numerous women under 25 who are also having symptoms and they are not allowed a smear test simply because of when they were born.'

But women with symptoms shouldn't and can't have what's classed as a screening test. If a woman has symptoms – bleeding after sex or in between periods, or offensive discharge or pain – she needs different tests. These wouldn't just be tests for cervical cancer (which could cause all of these symptoms) but tests for the bacterial infection chlamydia, and examination to look for vulval, cervical or vaginal conditions. Screening isn't for women with symptoms. Screening is for women who have no symptoms at all. If a woman with erratic bleeding after sex happens to have a negative smear test, that isn't enough to make us relax. She needs to be offered further tests to work out why.

The confusion means that some women with genital symptoms will think: 'Oh – it doesn't matter – my smear test was fine, so it can't be anything serious.' It may also mean that a woman thinks: 'Never mind – my smear is due in six months, I'll wait till then.' Screening tests can become a hook to hang our health fears on, but the coveted 'all clear' may be something of a false friend.

I have no doubt that some doctors struggle with this concept too, and I don't mean to pick on well meaning patient representatives. But getting this fundamental problem right is critical: if we don't accept the meaning, limitations and problems of screening, we are going to keep on getting it wrong.

5

Screening for more:
the prostate, bowel and aorta

Prostate cancer screening is never far from the media's bright lights. The subtext is this: women have their screening tests, so what about men? Don't they 'deserve' something to prevent their cancers, too?

It's a pity that these arguments are seldom advanced by balanced information that recognises that all screening comes with negatives attached. Dr Thomas Stuttaford, *The Times'* medical columnist for many years, was one of many campaigners for prostate cancer screening to be made available on the NHS.

The following is taken from an interview Stuttaford gave to the *BMJ* in 1998:

> '[Stuttaford] argues that the campaign for prostate cancer screening is justified. *The Times*, he suggests, has been right in the past about breast cancer and cervical cancer screening. "I can't think of when *The Times* has been wrong and the NHS has been right . . . You don't expect to see a reduction in mortality right away, because you're going to uncover the undiagnosed pool of prostate cancer."'[1]

The test Stuttaford wanted to see made widely available on the NHS is technically easier than either a smear or a mammogram. Instead, PSA – prostate-specific antigen – can be measured via a blood sample. It's relatively cheap, and can be repeated easily.

The problem with PSA is not with getting the test done; it's knowing what to do with the result.

Richard Ablin was the medical doctor at the University of Arizona who developed the PSA test in 1970. Doctors were looking for a way to track men who were known to have prostate cancer. PSA seemed to be a good way to see if men were responding to treatment. It wasn't completely reliable, but it could be used together with clinical examination, scans and symptoms to gauge how a man was getting on.

In 1986 PSA was approved by the US Food and Drug Administration for use in patients suspected of having prostate cancer; however, it started to be used frequently in North America as a screening test. A 'creep' set in.[2] The test wasn't just used when there was a suspicion of prostate cancer, but in men who were well and had no symptoms of disease.

Like so many very wrong things in medicine, screening for prostate cancer sounds beguiling, sensible, caring. Why wait until a man has symptoms of a disease that can kill him? Prostate cancer is the second most common cause of cancer death in men, after lung cancer. How could you deny men a potentially lifesaving simple little blood test?

At least, that's the way it has been framed by Stuttaford and his supporters. Many private clinics are eager to offer the test. Ablin, however, was horrified. He denounced the use of his PSA test as a screening test in *The New York Times* in 2010.

'. . . the test is hardly more effective than a coin toss. As I've been trying to make clear for many years now, PSA testing can't detect prostate cancer and, more important, it can't distinguish between the two types of prostate cancer – the one that will kill you and that one that won't . . .

I never dreamed that my discovery four decades ago would lead to such a profit-driven public health disaster. The medical community must confront reality and stop the inappropriate use of PSA screening.'[3]

Could Stuttaford have known in 1998 what Ablin pronounced in 2010? Probably. That's the problem with evidence – sometimes it tells you what you'd rather not know. Rather than assuming that early diagnosis was useful, we should have sought evidence right away. Rather than starting to screen men with it, doctors should have put the brakes on and insisted in only doing the test as part of a trial. Had we done this, we might have done far less damage to men.

By 1998, the journal *American Family Physician* was onto the problem of PSA testing and the evidence for harm – and lack of evidence for benefit. The journal had taken a deep breath and was telling us that, despite the American Cancer Society telling men over 50 to get the test:

> 'Data suggest that screening often detects what may be indolent, nonaggressive prostate cancer. The treatment of such a cancer with radiation or radical prostatectomy can result in significant morbidity, including urinary incontinence and impotence, without a proven decrease in mortality.'[4]

It's true. There is no point in identifying 'cancers' that will never harm a man. All you will do is give him pointless operations, radiotherapy and hormone therapy. The treatment for suspected prostate cancer includes surgery, with impotence as a potential side-effect. This might be fair enough should the choice be between impotence or death, but is it? Medicine entails a great deal of uncertainty, but without evidence to help patients call the odds, the doctor becomes a high stakes gambler. Of course, as a patient, you might not know this gamble is being made in your name.

Several major trials did then set out to reduce this uncertainty. These included RCTs, where one group of men was screened with the PSA test and another equal group was not. Some trials are still ongoing. One that found a benefit from PSA screening was the ERSPC study, the European Randomised Study of Screening for Prostate Cancer.[5] This followed 182,000 men aged between 55 and 69. In the screening group, 8.2% of men were diagnosed with prostate cancer over the course of the study, compared with 4.8% in the control group.

So more prostate cancer was diagnosed if men were screened with PSA tests. After almost nine years, there was a difference in death rates from prostate cancer between the groups. In the screening group (72,890 men), there had been 214 prostate cancer-related deaths by the end of the study. In the control group (89,353 men), 326 men had died from prostate cancer.

A success? In the screening group a lower percentage had died from prostate cancer – 0.29% in the screening group versus 0.36% in the control group.

But another way to look at the same numbers is with that way we came across earlier, the number needed to treat. The same numbers then tell you that 1,410 men had to be screened with PSA testing in order to stop one death from prostate cancer. This might seem okay – it's only a little blood test, after all. But men with a raised PSA went on to have further tests. This meant that 48 men needed to be treated for the raised PSA – biopsies, radiotherapy, surgery – for one man not to die from prostate cancer.

This might seem worthwhile to some men. Fair enough, but there are more studies to come, so don't make up your mind just yet. Before we get to them, there are two further problems with this study.

First, the study looked at prostate cancer deaths, not all deaths. But there's no point putting someone through the rigours of treatment for prostate cancer if the treatment causes a heart attack or a stroke, or the man was about to die from something else anyway. This may sound unbearably pessimistic, but it's true. If a patient is running the risk of surgery or anaesthesia there should be evidence that it's worth it. Do no harm, indeed. If we don't look for all-cause mortality – deaths no matter what was on the death certificate – we risk bias; we are not being 'holistic'. We should want to know what the chances are of life versus death – what goes on the death certificate is of secondary importance to the fact that it's being written at all. So we want to know about 'all-cause' mortality – will this test save life or reduce it?

The second issue is that this study included, under the banner of 'deaths from prostate cancer', any deaths that occurred due to treatment for prostate cancer. This is a problem because it may look like you died from prostate cancer when you died of unnecessary treatment, and this means bias. Let's look at another study, published in the same edition of the *NEJM* as the ERSPC study.

This separate study was part of the PLCO (Prostate, Lung, Colorectal and Ovarian) Cancer Screening Trial.[6] This study was done in the US, and contained almost 80,000 men, half of whom were given PSA testing over six years and half of whom were not. After ten years of follow-up, the researchers concluded that the death rate from prostate cancer was low and not very different between the two groups – in fact, there was even a slight rise in the deaths from prostate cancer in the men being screened. The findings contradicted the other study on PSA testing being reported in the same journal on the same day.

This study was a bit different in that it looked at what I like to see – all causes of death – not just prostate cancer. It did, though, report that seven years into the study, there were similar numbers of deaths from prostate cancer – 50 in the screening group and 44 in the control group. The important numbers are overall mortality. The authors say 'There was little difference between the two study groups in the number of deaths from other causes.' Overall, death rates in the two groups were much the same – slightly higher in the active screening group. We have no evidence from this study that more PSA testing can prolong your life.

This is what I mean about using all the available information, not just what suits your pet theory. These studies are just a couple of recent and high-profile ones on PSA testing. Digging back, there have been many fears that things were going badly wrong. An evidence update to the US Preventive Services Task Force in 2008 stated:

'Prostate cancer is the most common nonskin cancer in men in the United States, and prostate cancer screening has increased in recent years. In 2002, the US Preventive Services Task Force concluded that evidence was insufficient to recommend for or against screening for prostate cancer with prostate-specific antigen (PSA) testing. . . Few eligible studies were identified. Long term adverse effects of false positive PSA screening test results are unknown. Prostate-specific antigen screening is associated with psychological harms, and its potential benefits remain uncertain.'[7]

This is a subtly damning indictment of the culture of PSA screening. Despite doctors recommending, performing, interpreting and then acting on PSA screening test results, they had little evidence to back up what they were doing. In 2000, Dr Michael Barry in the *Journal of General Internal Medicine* referred to the 1990s as the 'PSA era' and said that the state of play in the 'evidence void' was 'nothing short of remarkable'.[8] Screening now resulted in an estimated overdiagnosis probability – the percentage of prostate cancers diagnosed by screening that would not have been diagnosed before death – of between 23% and 42%.[9]

Why were we in this mess? Some doctors had built their professional lives around PSA screening. They had everything to lose from denouncing – or even expressing doubts – about a test that was their bricks and mortar.

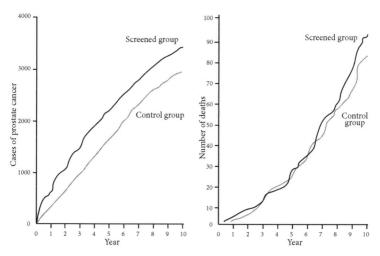

Mortality results from a randomized prostate-cancer screening trial.[6]

The origins of PSA

Thomas Stamey, a senior urologist from Stanford University School of Medicine, California, and colleagues published a paper in the *NEJM* in 1987 which led to the explosion of PSA testing worldwide. He compared PSA testing with another, then widely used, chemical, called PAP, prostatic acid phosphatase. He wanted to see which was the better chemical marker in men who had prostate cancer. He found that PSA was raised in 122 out of 127 newly diagnosed prostate cancer patients and that after removal of the prostate with surgery, the PSA level fell. The paper concluded that: 'PSA is more sensitive than PAP in the detection of prostate cancer and will probably be more useful in monitoring responses and recurrence after therapy.' It followed with the crucial sentence: 'However, since both PSA and PAP may be elevated in benign prostatic hyperplasia, neither marker is specific.'[10] So the test result would be elevated in any enlarged prostate gland, and since the prostate gland tends to enlarge over time, this means that normal men could have an abnormal result.

Somehow, intelligent people, who should have known far better, used this research to prompt them into running PSA levels on healthy men. Testing proliferated in private insurance schemes and, by 2000, Medicare in the US was offering PSA testing in all men over 50 years old, annually.[11] Heralding this advice, the US postal service stamped letters with the advice that men should have 'annual check-ups and tests'.[8]

But look at the flaws in transposing the information in Stamey's study to healthy men. Stamey's study didn't look at healthy men or how accurate or useful PSA was for detecting prostate cancer in them. The study didn't look at how precise the test was, or how PSA levels might vary in normal life. It was very far from looking at whether there was any advantage in having a screen-detected prostate cancer.

By the mid-1990s, several million PSA tests were being performed in the US each year. In the UK, testing for PSA more than doubled, from 1.4% of men aged 45 and over being screened in 1994, to 3.5% in 1999.[12]

Stamey and his colleagues did a brave thing. They examined just how well the PSA test results correlated to the cancer in the men they were screening in their practice. The tissue removed from 1,317 radical prostatectomies (complete removal of the prostate gland) performed in his unit over the previous 20 years was examined in detail by a pathologist. It turned out that the size and aggressiveness of tumours were not related to how high a PSA level was. Stamey concluded, in 2004, that:

'Serum PSA was related to prostate cancer 20 years ago. In the last five years serum PSA has only been related to benign prostatic hyperplasia.'

In other words, PSA was raised in men who didn't have cancer, but this is just the typical non-cancerous prostate enlargement (BPH, or benign prostatic hyperplasia) that goes along with ageing. But these screened men did end up having a major operation – a radical prostatectomy – which comes with the risk of impotence and incontinence. Autopsy information was instructive: prostate cancer is a very rare cause of death in young men, but since 31% of men over 50 who died of other causes had evidence of prostate cancer,[13] it is likely to be more common than we have anticipated – and often less harmful. Although Stamey said that 'our study raises a very serious question of whether a man should even use the PSA prostate cancer screening test any more',[14] the paper stated: 'What is urgently needed is a serum marker for prostate cancer that is truly proportional to the volume and grade of this ubiquitous cancer.'[15]

But we simply don't have that test.

Death with prostate cancer

It's well recognised that men can die with and not from prostate cancer. As far back as 1934, pathologists were writing to journals with the evidence of what they saw. For example, Arnold Rice Rich, MD, wrote in the *Journal of Urology*:

'For a number of years the writer has been impressed by the frequency with which small carcinomata have been found in the prostate in the routine autopsy material of this Department. It seems that these small tumours, which had attracted no attention clinically, and which were brought to light unexpectedly at autopsy, were being encountered much more often than the usual estimates of the frequency of occurrence of prostate carcinoma would have led one to expect.'[16]

Rich reported that a primary tumour – that is, a tumour starting in the prostate – was found in 14% of men over 50 who died from something else. That's a lot of men for whom having prostate cancer made no difference at all: they lived and died without even knowing they had it. If, though, it had been searched for, it would have been found. The men would have had gone through operations, chemotherapy and radiation therapy with no benefit to themselves, suffering all the inconvenience and side-effects for nothing; they were not going to die from prostate cancer.

What starts out as a logical train of action – prostate cancer is common and often silent, therefore screening would be useful – is usurped by complexities that could perhaps have been envisaged had we looked back far enough for all the evidence about prostate cancer with unbiased eyes.

The intentions of the doctors who started using PSA screening were honourable. But did they imagine what kind of problems PSA screening might dredge up? Did they even know enough about what prostate cancer is – and isn't?

I don't know. But if we had held back until we had researched the harms of screening just as much as its potential benefits, perhaps we wouldn't have generated the damaging fallout from PSA screening.

Selling PSA screening

Consider the tale told by two men, brothers who 'happened to be diagnosed with prostate cancer within a few months of one another'. This tale comes from the advertising blurb for a Harley Street clinic. The brothers had PSA testing done as a 'routine medical check-up'. Each proceeded to prostatic biopsy and then surgery, with 'the likely side-effects such as incontinence and erectile dysfunction'. One brother was only diagnosed because the treating doctor recommended that 'my two brothers would be well advised to have their PSA levels checked'. The second brother had been 'resisting family pressure to get his PSA test done for some time' but having had surgery, concludes:

> 'I suppose I should really have asked Roger Kirby why he wanted me to pen these reflections – apart from extolling the benefits of his treatment with the da Vinci machine [a robotic tool used in some prostate operations.] I am sure it was to encourage all men of my generation (50+) and especially those who, like me, tend to avoid anything medical, to ensure they have their PSA tested regularly. My medical check cost me hundreds of pounds – a PSA test can however be done on request free of charge at a GP's surgery. Bearing in mind we experienced absolutely no prior symptoms of our prostate cancers, both Jon and I consider ourselves the luckiest lads alive for having caught our conditions in good time – despite our delaying tactics!'[17]

This tale is recounted on the website of The Prostate Centre, a London clinic that says it 'lives and breathes men's health, and in particular everything that goes on around the prostate'.

The bottom line may be hard to accept if one has built a professional or personal life on prostate screening, but it is the bottom line nevertheless. We do not have good evidence that men with screen-detected prostate cancers do better than men who did not have the screening. They are, though, subjected to the physical, financial and emotional cost of patienthood. Is this a good deal for men?

Bowel cancer screening: it's new, but is it effective?

Most private health scanning clinics offer the option of screening for bowel cancer. Here there is an NHS crossover: a national screening programme for bowel cancer was started in 2006. Private scanning clinics tend to use bowel images, for example 'virtual colonoscopy' where the inside of the lower intestines can be viewed for signs of cancer. The NHS uses a different means, asking people aged between 60 and 69, and over that age on request, to take a sample of stool and send it on a specially prepared test strip to a laboratory. Here it is tested for faecal occult blood (FOB), which is blood in the stool that is invisible to the naked eye. Bleeding from the bowel can be a sign of bowel cancer. Coupled with the knowledge that bowel cancers frequently arise from polyps that can grow over years – even decades – before becoming cancerous, this simple test has, again, an enticing logic. Why not catch polyps before they turn into cancer?

By this stage in the evolution of screening, and possibly with some recognition of the problems that prostate, breast and cervical screening had produced, there was an intention to amass some evidence before starting a programme. The evidence accumulated from a pilot project – not a randomised controlled trial – performed in Scotland and England found that 1.9% of people screened had a positive test result. But the rate of detecting cancer was 0.16%. In other words, if you had a positive FOB test, you would only have cancer about 8% of the time. So in order to detect one cancer, 12.5 people would have to undergo further tests, usually a telescopic examination via the back passage, with biopsies being taken.[18] This is because an FOB test can be positive for lots of other reasons, from bleeding gums, to eating red meat, to piles – or just be a simply wrong result. FOB is not specific for bowel cancer.

Colonoscopy, the telescopic bowel test offered after a positive FOB screen, is about 90% accurate for picking up cancer. Colonoscopy can cause heavy bleeding after biopsy (one person in 150), perforation of the bowel (a 1 in 1,500 risk) or even death (a 1 in 10,000 risk.)[19] Even if you have a virtual test using a scanner and a polyp is seen or suspected, a biopsy, via colonoscopy, is usually needed for diagnosis.

We also need to know whether that test will lead to treatment that will delay death or be easier or more effective than later treatment. Bowel cancer is easier and better treated when it is contained in a polyp, rather than when it has spread. The more advanced the cancer, the more the need for chemotherapy and larger operations.

The NHS Bowel Screening Programme says that screening 'has been shown to reduce the risk of dying from bowel cancer by 16 per cent'. The reference for this is a Cochrane review, last assessed as being up to date in 2006.[20] But what does that mean? If you are given a 'relative risk' – here a 16% reduction in risk of dying from bowel cancer with screening – you need to know what your risk is to start off with. Relative risks tend to be impressive, sexier figures, but they can also be misleading.

A large risk factor for bowel cancer is increasing age. The Cochrane reviewers estimated that over ten years, the death rate for bowel cancer for males aged 40 and above, 50 and above, and 60 and above was 5, 22 and 70 respectively per 10,000 people.

With screening, they estimated that if the death rate could be reduced by 16% the mortality rates from bowel cancer would fall to 4.2, 18.5, and 58.8 for the respective age groups, again per 10,000 population.

Certainly, that's a reduction. If millions of people took part, that could tot up to an impressive dent in bowel cancer figures. But to get that dent, you have to put a colonoscope into the bowels of many more people than actually have cancer. The screening process is not risk free. So if you are 60 years old, screening will reduce your risk of dying with bowel cancer from 70 to 58.8 per 10,000 population – a reduction in absolute risk from 0.7% to 0.58%.

This doesn't look quite the same as the 'reduction in death rate by 16%' we were promised in the blurb. Here's another really important point made in the same Cochrane review:

> 'Combining the four trials did not show any significant difference in all-cause mortality between the screening and control groups.'

It's important, so important, to look at the bigger picture: are we offering people more years of life with screening – or are some of the benefits of earlier diagnosis negated through the consequences of the treatment people are offered? Certainly, even if there were no gain to life length with a screening programme it could still be useful to offer it. There could be other advantages to screening: for example, smaller, easier operations could perhaps be offered; quality of life, if not quantity, might be improved. But do we know this? We don't. We have not proven that bowel screening results in longer lives.

So what do we do? Bowel cancer screening cuts deaths from bowel cancer, but there is no evidence for it increasing life length overall: it comes with false positives and false negatives, and some risk, albeit small, of harms arising from the consequences of screening.

Do we even get to know that these challenging and complex decisions need to be made? We do not. We get the sizzle of advertising from public as well as private sectors, playing on our anxieties and then offering to soothe our nerves if our scans are normal, or find problems 'early' if they are not.

As for whether or not you are more likely or less likely to be spared major surgery if diagnosed with bowel cancer at colonoscopy, I cannot say. So far the evidence around screening has focused on gathering mortality and morbidity data. The stitch-in-time theory of having a polypectomy now rather than a major operation later may be valid if, for example, you have a strong family history of bowel polyps. Otherwise, we are left with a lot of questions.

Assessing the aorta

Life Line Screening, which we've noted offers private health checks, often in local church halls, also offers ultrasound examinations of the aorta, the main artery in the abdomen. According to its leaflet:

> 'A painless ultrasound examination, like that used on expectant mothers, is used to screen for the presence of an aneurysm in the abdominal aorta that could lead to a ruptured aortic artery . . .

if we find a condition that requires immediate attention, we will notify you on the day of the screening so that you can consult your GP immediately.'

This major artery from the heart to the lower body, the aorta, can indeed develop aneurysms. These balloonings of the shape of the normally straight artery may cause no bother, no symptoms and no complications. But they can also rupture. This can be fatal. It can happen suddenly, without warning, and require major emergency surgery.

Ideally, if you need to have major surgery, you want to plan it as much as possible. You want to have blood cross-matched and ready for you if you need a transfusion. You want a bed with your name on it booked in intensive care. You want an anaesthetist who knows your blood pressure and any medication that you're on, and you want a chance to lose weight, give up smoking and be as fit as possible before going near a hospital bed.

Emergency surgery is altogether riskier. You may need it when you are miles away from a hospital, for a start. You may be unwell for other reasons, be rushed to theatre with no cross-matched blood ready and no surgeon nearby who specalises in what you currently need – that is, a fast plumbing job to the major blood vessel in your body. You may have already lost blood, and blood pressure, by the time you get to the operating table.

Thus, given the option, you'd choose to be operated on in a planned, controlled, and organised manner. On the face of it, that's what finding an aortic aneurysm at a check-up seems to offer. It may be bad news, but the idea is that you have a chance to deal with it in the best circumstances possible.

In 2010, the NHS started the roll-out of just such a screening programme. It targets men aged 65 for a one-off ultrasound scan, saying that it 'could reduce the rate of premature death from ruptured AAA (abdominal aortic aneurysm) by up to 50%'.[21]

As before: what exactly does that 50% mean?

The NHS information tells us the following: there are 6,000 deaths per year from ruptured AAA in England and Wales, and 2% of men aged over 65 die of it.[21] So the NHS's new screening programme is offering to cut the death rate from 6,000 to 3,000.

Impressive. So what does it cost? The scheme is organised so that men with no, or a very small, aneurysm will be scanned once and discharged from the programme. Men with aneurysms between 3cm and 5.4cm wide will be offered repeat scans, either yearly or three-monthly. Men with aneurysms greater than 5.5cm are referred directly to a vascular surgeon for a discussion about a major operation.

But what's the cost? I don't mean pounds and pence. What side-effects and other adverse consequences do we have to accept in order to cut the death rate for AAA so dramatically?

First, is it so dramatic at all? Perhaps not. The origin of the '50% cut' in AAA deaths is a big, randomised, multi-centred study containing almost 70,000 men. It was published in the *BMJ* in 2009, complete with a little box highlighting and emphasising its wonder: 'About half of all aneurysm-related deaths should be prevented by a national screening programme.'[22]

Yet half of a small number is an even smaller number. Instead of relative risk, we need to know the absolute risk (notice a pattern?) How many AAA deaths can we prevent with screening?

Over ten years, in the screened group of 33,883 men, there were 155 deaths related to AAA. In the control group of 33,887 men, there were 296 deaths related to AAA.

Look at this another way: 0.46% of men in the screened group died of AAA. In the unscreened, control group, 0.87% of men died of AAA. In absolute terms, this is a reduction in deaths of 0.41%.

What else? Again, we want to know overall mortality. Planned surgery is less risky than emergency surgery, but any surgery is more risky than none. That's not a dig at surgeons and anaesthetists. There is never no risk.

In AAA screening, it's the choice between doing something (an operation that you may or may not benefit from, and which you may or may not recover speedily from) and doing nothing (ignoring the results or not having a scan, which, again, may or may not benefit you). Did you delay your death from AAA, or not?

What I want, in true broken record style, is the all-cause mortality. There is little point not dying of an AAA thanks to major preventive surgery, only to die of a heart attack as you are recovering.

Here are the numbers for all-cause mortality, ten years into the same multicentre study. In the control group, there were 10,481 deaths. In the screening group, there were 10,274 deaths. The vast majority were nothing to do with aneurysms. In percentage terms, within the control group, 30.93% of the men died; in the screened group, 30.32% of the men died.

Yes, there's a difference. But it is small. Is it fair on a man considering whether or not to have one of these scans to tell him that it will reduce his risk of dying of an AAA by half?

There are other considerations. How risky is an elective, planned repair of an AAA?

This has been answered by several studies that have examined how likely you are to die after a planned AAA repair. They found that age, male sex, cardiac disease and diabetes were risk factors for death and that the mortality rate (at 28 days in men post-surgery) varied from 3.3% to 27.1%, according to age.[23] An English study published in 2000 suggested that the mortality rate from elective (planned) repair was around 7%.[24] A further study from the UK found that men diagnosed with an AAA at screening had a post-operative mortality rate that was lower, at 6%.[25]

In terms of operation risk, a risk of death of around one in 20 is relatively high. Most routine operations don't carry this mortality rate. While some factors, like using surgeons who are specialised in treating AAA, can help improve survival rates, there is always going to be risk. The same vascular disease that contributed to the aneurysm formation may mean vascular disease elsewhere, particularly the heart.

What happens to men who are told that, either they have an aneurysm not yet big enough for surgery but may require it in the future, or that they have an AAA but co-existing medical problems such as heart disease make them too high risk to consider an operation. What then?

There has been some consideration of the psychological

consequences of AAA screening but my questions remain unanswered. A well-known depression and anxiety score, the HADS questionnaire – basically ticking boxes about how you are feeling – has been used to compare men who have and haven't been screened. It compared men with small aneurysms having follow-up, men awaiting surgery and men who had normal scans with men who hadn't been screened. Similar scores were found.

But this isn't telling me quite enough. Men who have been screened and told they are 'normal' may be feeling reassured, less anxious and perhaps better than usual. The effect of these men may balance out an adverse effect on other, less fortunate men – so is it fair to conclude that there are no appreciable psychological side-effects? Men who were told they had an aneurysm but were too 'risky' for surgery were not specifically addressed.[26]

As a GP, I can often fall back on research to guide me when I am doing something I'd rather not be doing – overseeing crying children being vaccinated, for example. I don't like to see children upset but I know that these children will not see measles kill them or their siblings, as happens every day in many underdeveloped countries where vaccination is not carried out.

So when a man comes into my surgery who is devastated by his AAA screening result, and who has been told it is too risky to operate, I'd like to be able to rationalise the 'adverse psychological consequences' in a way that makes me feel that the right thing has been done. If someone was always going to be unfit for surgery, was there any point in screening him, finding an AAA, and then saying that there was nothing to be done but wait and see? I find that cruel.

The problem with studying groups, as we do, is that it is easy to miss the story of an individual. As a GP, I am biased: it is individuals, and families containing individuals, who I see, and it is my job to help each person to measure positives and negatives, the random and unforeseen with the predictable and difficult.

My professional experience has taught me always to act with care; something that might not make one person blink might make another think about writing their will.

And the church hall?

Oh yes. The UK Vascular Society has been beavering away, asking vexing and difficult questions like: Who should we screen? When? How often? Others, though, have dispensed with such uncertainties.

The Life Line Screening website is full of thrusting, earnest advice about the company's 'health screening services'. For AAA screening, it says:

'Because AAA are likely to tear if they reach 5 centimeters in diameter, monitoring is important to prevent rupture. A ruptured AAA can cause blood loss, shock and death. Life Line Screening uses ultrasound technology to measure the size of your abdominal aorta. The process is painless . . .'

Most AAAs do not rupture, and it is not merely the ultrasound that will prevent you dying from an AAA. Unlike the NHS, which recognises that a one-off screening will at least find a big group of men who have no AAA and are thus very unlikely to develop one and die of it, Life Line Screening just says:

'How often should you get screened? This is a personal decision based on your risk factors and previous screening results. Many of our customers have an annual screening as part of their regular healthcare regime.'[27]

But reducing a death rate from ruptured AAA via a screening programme involves major surgery: you need to know that before you start unbuttoning your shirt.

6

Health for sale: everyone wants a slice of the healthy patient

Well people are the health marketeer's dream. It's not just screening tests that are sold to healthy people. There is a low-level, insidious grind of health advertising attempting to persuade well people that they need to buy into their healthcare.

I shop to find good things to eat and drink, and this should be fun. Instead, I have to step around aisles that are full of health alerts. Cholesterol – vital to our body, required for healthy brain and nerves – is a particular bête noire of twenty-first century nutrition. You may have heard smooth-voiced celebrities murmuring the wonders of cholesterol-lowering margarine on the radio, or seen the red flashes on margarine labels telling you of the 'scientific evidence' that proves these spreads lower cholesterol. And they're right; these spreads do lower cholesterol.

In fact, if you ask the manufacturers of Benecol, one of the 'cholesterol-lowering' spreads, they will claim that there is 'a wealth of evidence demonstrating the efficacy of plant stanols in the reduction of total and LDL (bad) cholesterol levels'. The makers of Flora, another similar margarine, cite 'over 140 studies to show that plant sterols reduce cholesterol and over 40 studies to show that Flora pro.activ spread specifically reduces cholesterol'.[1]

So what's my problem? I really want to know whether or not the lowering of cholesterol via our shopping basket is just an interesting laboratory finding or whether it pays out in real life. Does using this margarine regularly either stop us from having as many heart attacks and strokes, or allow us to live longer?

The Flora website tells us that eating '1.5g to 2.4g of plant sterols daily can lower LDL cholesterol by 7-10% in 2-3 weeks.'[2] This means three portions of their spread, or one of their 'mini drinks', which contain these sterols. But I don't really want to know whether or not this margarine will make a dent in my cholesterol.

Why? The biggest and best studies that have examined the effects of lowering cholesterol over years – such as the WOSCOPS study,[3] performed in the heart attack-prone west of Scotland – concentrated on using statin tablets to get the numbers down. There are no large studies that show that lowering cholesterol through using dairy products will either stop a stroke or delay your death.

Some people might argue that this doesn't matter. If studies show that lowering cholesterol is good for you, what does it matter if the mechanism of getting there is different, and we do it by diet instead of tablets?

Here we get into the tricky 'proxy outcome' problem. The best-known of the major studies looking at the effect of cholesterol on health is the Framingham series of studies, which has collected data about the several thousand residents of this town in Massachusetts, USA, since 1971. The research has extended to the children of original study members and has spawned hundreds of frequently cited scientific papers. Many routes to work out the future risk of a person having a heart attack or stroke here in the UK are largely based on Framingham data.[4]

Framingham data tell us that having a high LDL cholesterol was associated with a higher risk of heart attack and stroke, and that having a high HDL level was associated with a lower risk of heart attack and stroke.

It's important to be clear about what 'associated' means here. The original Framingham study was about 'observing'. The researchers found that higher or lower levels of the types of cholesterol seemed to lead to different outcomes. They didn't explain why that was, or whether you could prevent deaths through lowering cholesterol.

So further studies were needed to try to work out what deliberately lowering cholesterol levels would do. This couldn't be done with an observational study, but needed an interventional study. Many, many of these studies have now been done. Mainly, they involve giving some participants in the trial a cholesterol-lowering drug, usually a statin. The best studies are randomised and placebo controlled, so that the members of the group (and the researchers, too, if it's 'double' blind, see box) don't know who is getting the real or dummy tablets. This minimises bias and means you can be more certain about your results. By comparing what happens next, you can work out if the 'real' tablets are having an effect – or not. If you can show that the 'real tablets' are the only difference between the two groups, you can be more sure that any difference in heart attacks between the groups is down to the

Blinded studies

Double blind study – neither patients nor researchers know which patients get what intervention. For example, the patient and researcher don't know whether the tablets are placebo or have active ingredients until the trial is over.

Single blind study – the researcher knows which treatment each patient gets, but the patients don't know. For example, the patient may not know the type of operation done under anaesthetic by the surgeon, who must know. This may be problematic if the researcher has to make an assessment of the patient's improvement, because it can create bias.

Unblinded study – here both patient and researcher know what intervention is being done. Because of this, this kind of study carries a higher risk of bias.

ingredient in the pills.

Some of those type of studies are quite famous. WOSCOPS showed that cholesterol-lowering tablets reduced the rate of heart attack and stroke in men without a history of cardiovascular disease. The '4S' study (Scandinavian Simvastatin Survival Study) looked at the effect of statins in people who had heart disease, and agreed about the benefits.[5] In both these studies, it was the statin that made the difference, pulling towards the conclusion that it was these pills that had the effect.

The margarine manufacturers want to piggyback on this research: if lowering cholesterol with statins is good, then lowering it with margarine is also good. But while the margarine might lower cholesterol, we don't know if that will reduce the rate of heart attacks or strokes, since there are no studies to prove it. This is skipping a research step or two: relying on what are called 'proxy outcomes'. The manufacturers choose to assume that lowering cholesterol with margarine will have the same effect as lowering cholesterol with statins.

Relying on proxy outcomes adds an extra layer of uncertainty to our uncertainties. What we need is a trial, just like WOSCOPS or 4S, to establish whether margarine makes a difference. We don't have that – there is no massive margarine study showing that slathering it on muffins stops heart attacks or strokes.

Running studies costs time and money; using proxy outcomes is cheap and fast. Who wants to fund long-term studies of margarine use when you can hitch your wagon to already established research?

The Flora website has a section aimed at professionals – with Clooneyesque doctors gazing thoughtfully from their missives. In a document entitled 'Plant sterol-enriched foods clinically proven to lower cholesterol', we are told that there are 'more than 180 studies' in support of this thesis.[6] However, most involve a small number of patients, and none uses things like mortality or morbidity as outcomes.[7] More poor-quality studies do not mean better proof.

The bottom line is that we don't know if using these products will save your life – or, to be more accurate, delay your death.

What those flashes on margarine packets should really say is 'Proven to lower cholesterol a bit. Not proven to independently lower risk of heart attack or stroke. Buyer beware!' Personally, I'd also add that it doesn't taste as good as butter, but that's just me.

Health, happiness and yogurt

'Our mission is to bring health through food & beverages to a maximum number of people in the UK' says Danone, a manufacturer of yogurts, artificial milk and bottles of water. The company's European website claims that 'Not only does your pot a day taste fabulous, it's also a little wonder pot of goodness for your tummy!'[8] On Danone's sister website 'Probiotics in Practice', designed for healthcare professionals, it claims that 'Probiotics are meanwhile widely acknowledged by scientists and healthcare professionals to exert beneficial effects that support health and wellbeing.'[9]

Is this true? Danone's clinical studies page cites four studies under the heading 'digestive comfort', conducted in people with either this complaint or 'irritable bowel syndrome' (IBS).[10] Let us run through them.

The first was a decent kind of study,[11] a randomised trial, comparing women taking two portions of ordinary yogurt a day, or a yogurt without the bacterial strain in it. At week four, they had an 'overall assessment of gastrointestinal well-being'; 41% had improved in the live yogurt group versus 34% in the control group: therefore, seven people in 100 taking this yogurt were getting a benefit from it (because 34 in 100 got better anyway.) This number of people who got better with the placebo (normal) yogurt alone is important, because digestive symptoms tend to wax and wane, and can appear to get better because of a treatment when really, the treatment had no effect. The symptoms were likely to improve anyway.

The second study was weaker. It was an open-label study, which means that participants would be aware of whether or not they were taking the placebo yogurt – which came in branded tubs. In this case, more than 82% of people got better when taking the 'live' yogurt compared with just 2.9% improving with placebo.[12] Does this mean the live yogurt works? No – the researchers, who acknowledged this was simply a pilot study, also said that 'double blind randomised controlled trials are required to confirm these health benefits'. Isn't it interesting that blinding – not telling the participants what was in the bottle – resulted in little improvement, but unblinding them – telling them what they were getting – resulted in a big improvement?

Study number three was randomised and blinded – the participants didn't know whether or not they were getting the 'active' yogurt.[13] The 34 patients who took part charted their symptoms. Let's look at the symptoms of irritable bowel syndrome (IBS), since this is what the stuff is really being marketed for – the on-and-off symptoms of loose or constipated bowel movements and cramping pain, often related to stress or anxiety. The two groups scored their symptoms on a chart. In the active yogurt group, the average symptom score – where 5 is the highest – was 3.3 versus a score of 3.8 for the control group. However, the starting scores – before any yogurt was imbibed – were 3.7 for the active group and 3.9 for the control group. Not much of a difference at all. Sure, the study collected other data as well – transit time through the bowel and waist measurements – but I'm interested in what the people taking the stuff actually felt. And the answer is not much at all.

The final study? This was a randomised controlled trial on adults with predominantly constipation-type IBS.[14] Again, let's look at the pattern of symptoms over the six-week course of this trial. The participants were asked to score their symptoms at the end of six weeks. The total number of participants in the trial was 19, and there were large differences in the symptoms scores between the participants before the trial was started, making them appear unmatched. Again, differences between scores after the trial were small and of questionable real-life benefit.

Thus the results, if you discount the trial that wasn't randomised and blinded, are not impressive. They do not promise any huge improvements to people with abdominal pain from IBS. Yet Danone insists that its products are 'good for digestive health'.

Very suspect vitamins

At least Danone actually did some trials. Without trials, you have little idea about what the effects of your interventions are. Take, for example, Vitaminwater, a product made by Coca-Cola. This luridly coloured drink is widely available and advertised using slightly camp slogans: 'More muscles than brussels', 'Keep perky when you're feeling murky' and 'Vitamin C and zinc to help you spend less time reading old magazines in the doctor's waiting room'.

The comment on the quality of magazines in our waiting room bridled – we always have pretty good reading material. But what disturbed me even more was the sight of a dear and very intelligent friend clutching a bottle of Vitaminwater. I grabbed it out of his hand, and read the label.

The sugar content in a single 500ml bottle is 23g – a quarter of your total recommended daily sugar allowance. That was what made me complain; there was a national advertising campaign but only a couple of other people in the whole of the UK joined me in voicing objections to the Advertising Standards Authority. Apathy in these matters might be fair enough, since the whole thing appeared so silly, but the adverts edged into medical territory by claiming that the vitamins in the drink would act as some kind of 'defense' – the ASA said the company was 'claiming that the products could increase resistance to illness'.[15]

Just a daft, misleading advertising campaign? The advertisers were tapping into the belief that vitamins are good for us. This view is propagated by many health food shops and pharmacies, where we can find vitamins and supplements in packaging shining with confident smiles.

But vitamins are good for us, aren't they? Alas, just because there are thousands of these products on sale doesn't mean that this is true.

Lots of evidence points out that eating a diet rich in fruit and vegetables, grains and pulses will result in a longer, better quality life. Proxy outcomes alert! The proxy says: Fruit and vegetables are healthy. Vitamins are in fruit and vegetables. Therefore vitamins are healthy. Vitamins are good for us.

But it's counterintuitive. Research has told us a fair bit about vitamin supplements. We know that folic acid, one of the vitamin B group, taken prenatally and during the first three months of pregnancy, can reduce the rate of spinal cord deformities in newborn babies.[16] We have evidence that vitamin A and zinc supplements can reduce illness and improve death rates in HIV-infected women and children.[17] But these are special groups. What about non-pregnant people with no immune problems? Can vitamins really make us feel better or be more healthy?

Alas, medicine, as we have found, does not always fit with what sounds logical and reasonable. From the very first surgeons who believed that bloodletting was a good way to let out all your bad humours, what seems sensible at the time is only ever built on our contemporary understanding. It's fantastically easy to see only what you want to. So, in mediaeval barber shops, if people bled to death, they were going to die anyway. Nothing to do with that scarlet puddle on the floor. If someone got better, though, they had been saved by the bloodletting. It's easier to ignore the other explanation that only the fittest managed to survive the 'treatment'.

Some research has been reported as saying that a deficiency of vitamins causes cancer. Indeed, there is a lot of research about antioxidants, which mop up 'free radicals' – unstable molecules created during the normal workings of the body's cells – which can build up, cause cellular damage and increase the risk of cancer. The antioxidant vitamins, E, C and beta carotene – a vitamin A precursor – would appear to be the logical thing to take to prevent these free radicals from accumulating and hence prevent cancer from developing.

At least, that's the highly plausible reasoning you may encounter at shops selling them. A better question would be: what happens when healthy people take regular vitamins? Do they get less cancer? No, is the short answer. Not a shy, coy, uncertain 'no' but an emphatic, evidence-based 'no'. Here is the conclusion from a Cochrane review, which, let's recall, is a review that takes account of all the evidence, not just the agreeable highlights:

'There is currently no evidence to support recommending vitamins such as alpha-tocopherol (vitamin E), beta-carotene or retinol (vitamin A) alone or in combination, to prevent lung cancer. A harmful effect was found in beta-carotene with retinol at pharmacological doses in people with risk factors for lung cancer (smoking and/or occupational exposure to asbestos).'[18]

This needs a bit of a double-take, because it is, again, counterintuitive. The very people who were at higher risk of getting lung cancer actually did worse when they took anti-oxidants, with an increase in lung cancer diagnosed – although there was no change in overall death rates between smokers who took vitamins and smokers who didn't.

It's not what we expect to find. It's also annoying – we would like a nice vitamin tablet to give nicotine addicts to stop them getting cancer.

People who want to prove a point will often be able to find some bit of research or other that they can use to support it. If you look at the PubMed website, which lists medical research, you will find millions of papers. An important part of reducing uncertainty about good treatments is that you are able to replicate your research. It's not good enough to find that homoeopathy worked in a small collection of patients, once. You want to make sure that you can reliably repeat your findings and replicate them elsewhere. Citing just one study that says vitamins are great might also mean that you are ignoring the findings of 50 other studies that say the opposite. The fairest way is to look at all the evidence before judging what works.

In other words, Cochrane. In 2010 the Cochrane Collaboration looked at all the evidence, meticulously sifting and gathering evidence about vitamin use in healthy people. The researchers noted that there was animal research indicating that vitamins improved mortality rates. They noted that there was a theoretical reason to consider that vitamins could be a good thing. They found a total of 67 trials, with 232,550 participants, asking that question. And they found no evidence that antioxidants improved health in people who were completely healthy, or even in people who already had a disease.[19]

Boots is a massive high street presence. Where supermarkets have alluring sweeties beside the till, Boots has a variety of pills, often vitamin supplements, and usually on special '3 for 2' offer. Boots Probiotic says it 'helps maintain a healthy immune system', while its Feel the Difference multivitamins for women claim to 'support the female body'. The best nonsense though is Boots Feel the Difference Instant Vitality Vitamin C and Probiotic. 'Instant vitality'? Please.

We don't get good enough information at the point of sale that helps us decide, rationally, if this stuff will do us any good or not. But adverts for vitamins, margarine, and yogurt are minnows compared with the other health juggernauts intent on turning perfectly well people into patients.

Predicting pregnancy

Infertility can be distressing as well as difficult to manage. Most couples – around 90% – will achieve pregnancy within a year, and a few more percent in the years after that.[20] Clearly, the majority of couples having regular sex are not going to need fertility aids or treatments as the vast majority will get pregnant by themselves.

So why is there an industry targeted at couples who are at the beginning, or have not yet even started, to try for pregnancy?

The Babystart company, for example, offers tests for predicting when ovulation will take place, as well as a 'fertility screening test for both men and women'.[21] The latter includes a home test for follicle-stimulating hormone (FSH) in women, which varies naturally during a normal menstrual cycle, only rising consistently when a woman stops menstruating and enters menopause. The male test, a sperm count, offers an alert if the result falls below the World Health Organization criteria for sperm concentration. In small print, the company does say the test 'is not proof of fertility'. Too right.

The only fertility test that really counts is having sex. There is no test that you can do of your fertility that will guarantee that you can conceive and give birth to a child. As many as 15% of infertile couples have 'unexplained' infertility, which is when all tests on each partner are returned as being 'normal'.[22] Many men whose tests show subfertile levels of sperm will later be shown to have higher levels; simple viral infections like colds or flu can temporarily reduce supply. But what actually matters? A study published in the *NEJM* in 2001 noted that what the WHO used to call 'normal' sperm values were now classed as 'reference' values because it was so difficult to decide where normal and abnormal lay. These researchers compared semen samples of infertile and fertile men, and found an overlap of results. They concluded that:

> 'None of the measures, alone or in combination, can be considered diagnostic of infertility. . . . our data suggest that caution must be used in interpreting the significance of any given subfertile or indeterminate semen measurement. Although low values for each measurement increase the likelihood that a male factor contributes to infertility, there was substantial overlap in the frequency distributions in our study.'[23]

The amount and type of sperm you need to conceive is not, therefore, as simple as a straightforward testing kit would have you believe. So what happens when men test themselves and find a 'low' reading? If you believe the sales pitch, these men are to feel glad that a problem is being picked up quickly. But what if it isn't a problem; what if natural conception is likely to follow? Sadly, I find that many couples are made distressed and anxious at a time when they should be excited about their future. This little test might not help them but instead turn their happiness to misery and worry.

The fertility market is burgeoning. Zita West, a midwife who says that she has 'unrivalled experience in helping couples who are finding it difficult to get pregnant' offers a 'five star start to life' in her approach to getting couples pregnant.[24] 'Want to know how fertile you are?' she asks. 'The relatively new anti-Mullerian hormone (AMH) test is thought to be the most accurate predictor of a woman's ovarian reserve and is the basic test that we would usually recommend if a woman wanted to check on her fertility status.' She offers results expressed as 'optimal', 'satisfactory', 'low' or 'very low/undetectable'. In fact, she offers the same test to women who 'want to plan ahead', are unsure whether their 'fertility is where it needs to be', may have been trying to conceive for a while, or who may be thinking about IVF.[25]

Yet none of this reflects the realistic situation that couples may find themselves in. If you want reassurance that you can delay pregnancy until you are ready, this test isn't it; your test can be 'optimal', but all it measures is the ovarian reserve, not how open the fallopian tubes are, how receptive the womb is or how able the sperm are. This test could be entirely reassuring but pregnancy may still be difficult to achieve, while even if the test is lower than 'optimal', a woman may still find it relatively easy to become pregnant. If a couple are not conceiving, this test is not necessary, but others may be: knowing the other female hormone levels would be useful as would male tests. This is why the Royal College of Obstetricians and Gynaecologists published a book called *Reproductive Ageing*, in which it says that the value of this AMH test 'in predicting clinically relevant outcomes (pregnancy and live birth) is either poor or unknown'.[26] The only test of getting pregnant is having sex. The idea that one can provide a reliable prediction of a future happy event is simply unrealistic.

In fact, the AMH test was developed not to measure future fertility, but to help plan treatment in women who had known fertility problems, for example, those whose treatment for cancer was likely to result in infertility. This had dovetailed with research trying to predict which women with (known) infertility were going to do well with IVF. This is an entirely different set-up to a woman who just wants a 'check'.

In fact, an 'optimal' test result might actually be harmful. If a woman believes that she has adequate ovarian 'reserve' she may delay pregnancy for months or years. Yet the very best predictor of successful pregnancy is not AMH but age. The older a woman, the less likely she is to have a healthy pregnancy and live birth. And the older a woman is, the less successful are treatments for infertility.

Zita West is not alone in offering 'Fertility MOTs'. Most cities entertain companies offering them, and many private hospital chains also offer a specific testing session.[27] Competitions for a 'free fertility check' launched at least one private hospital's new enterprise. One press report featured a woman who was surprised, at the age of 37, to be told that her fertility rate was falling and to 'get a move on' by the doctor. In fact, the advice that fertility is highest in the 20s and falls in the mid-30s would have been the same whether or not she had any (expensive) tests at all.[28]

The bigger question is whether relying on medical tests for an answer stops us looking at the more complex reality. Fertility cannot be guaranteed. Fertility falls with age. Having sex to attempt pregnancy is the only true test of fertility. Obscuring or diffusing these facts with questionable tests does not help.

The cervical cancer jab

'It's amazing', gushes a pharmacist, on one of Boots' promotional videos. 'It's a vaccination that helps you stop catching human papilloma virus . . . if customers are interested they can come instore or telephone.' And: 'Cervical cancer is a really important cancer to treat. . . We can also help people understand the importance of their smear tests.'[29]

To which I say: no, no, no.

Cervical cancer certainly is important to treat. But the pharmacist is not talking about the treatment of cervical cancer, she is talking about trying to prevent it by using the HPV (human papilloma virus) vaccination – and doing so outside the current NHS recommendations, which are to offer it to girls aged 12 and 13.

The HP virus causes most cervical cancers. Most women get infected with HPV. But most women do not get cervical cancer – their own immunity clears the HPV from the cervical cells.[30] The logic is that immunising young people before they are sexually active – hence before they are exposed to HPV – will prevent them being infected.

But does it work? Yes, say the manufacturers, who have shown that the vaccine is very effective against two types of HPV, 16 and 18, which cause 70% of cervical cancers. They launched the vaccine citing two large randomised trials that showed a decrease in cervical cellular changes or localised cancer three years after treatment.[31,32] And thus the NHS adopted their vaccination programme.

The vaccine may be safe enough – it has been closely monitored – but is it effective? We don't know what will happen to the virus: if subtypes numbers 16 and 18 are being defeated, shall we, over time, see an upsurge in other variants of the virus? Will HPV vaccination make people less likely to use barrier forms of contraception, which also protect against other types of sexual infection? Is the immunity to HPV long lasting or should the vaccination be repeated? Would the vaccine work if it was repeated, just as rubella vaccine can be repeated, if immunity wears down over time? The 'Future' trial[32] included women who had had no more than four sexual partners; the 'Patricia' trial[31] allowed six partners. Is this relevant?

The NHS vaccination campaign has been rolled out without answers to these questions. It would be ludicrous to stop doing anything new in healthcare until we knew absolutely everything about it – but when there are big uncertainties, we have to acknowledge them and make sure they are accounted for. This would normally be done by using the new intervention in trials or audit, so that you could track what was happening and ensure that intervention was effective and useful. Boots is using the vaccine in a different way. In people who have had sex, and may have been exposed to HPV, it doesn't work well. Once you've been exposed to the virus, you will not get the same immunity from vaccination. To be effective, it has to be given before exposure – through sex – to HPV. In studies that have looked at the vaccination in sexually active women, it is far less efficient in reducing cervical cell changes.[33] Do women get warned about this lack of effectiveness before handing over almost £300 to Boots? There is no warning about this or comparison to the NHS recommendations on the company's website.

In every example of a health intervention being offered to a healthy person, there are problems. There are questions. Difficulties. Pros and cons. People will have different priorities and want to make different choices – making decisions about health based on false promise and unfair lure is not a fair choice.

'False promise and unfair lure' of course, could happily sum up rather a lot of advertising. But the very nature of adverts – short, snappy, memorable – runs counter to the ethos of making sound medical decisions. These, by nature, take longer, require analytical skills and need to factor in the person's own priorities, background and concerns.

Sexed-up medicine, public and private health

Where does this leave us, doctors and citizens, meeting the new and extending outreach of medicine? Fifty years ago, the screening agenda didn't exist. People who were well were left alone. Blood pressures, cholesterols, cervixes and bowels went unexamined unless the patient had symptoms suggesting a problem. You and your family were usually known at your doctor's surgery. If you were well, you were well, and you were mainly unhindered with messages of what to do, eat or take to assure your health. Public health doctors made sure that clean water and, later, immunisations were available to all who needed them. Otherwise, you did not hear much from medicine. It stood at a respectful distance and left you alone.

That clear distinction between patient and person no longer exists. Citizens are now urged to undergo screening tests either to confirm a state of non-illness, or predict risk of early death or disease. Because 'no risk' does not exist, we never get complete assurance that we are well. If a screening test shows, instead, a low risk of disease, we are encouraged to make a date for our next screening test, reminded of what we should do to stay 'healthy', and what we should worry about in the meantime. Scoring systems for cardiovascular risk or screening for conditions like depression make us more likely to overdiagnose problems and treat people who will not benefit from that treatment. As we have seen, modern medicine's new victims are people who are labelled with illness or risk or treated with medical drugs or interventions although they will never benefit from them.

Some people think this to be fair enough, a reasonable exchange, and one worth making. Sure, but just as people should be free to choose that gamble, others should be free not to.

We do not live – thankfully – in a society where we are treated as sheep, led to feed on medicine when and where instructed. We expect – do we not? – to be involved in deciding what to do with our bodies.

Hard-sell, sexed-up medicine does not give us that free choice. Because the information we are given is chosen to lead us, not inform us, we don't get fair information. Rather than GPs working for the individual in front of them, through screening and risk management they have taken on the devolved duty of the public health physician. Because some things might be good for populations, family doctors have been pushed into applying the same principles of population health to individual people.

This is a fundamental loss to both patients and GPs. It's here that the patient paradox starts to create moral, ethical and scientific dilemmas; as we will see, this is the start of medicine going badly wrong.

PART TWO

The way it works

7

George Clooney and the medical certainty illusion

You've been advertised to, hooked and drawn in – what next? What happens when you relinquish personhood and become a patient? If we take the opportunity of screening, testing and measuring, we risk becoming patients, so we should know how it works behind the scenes.

It's all (at least) a little bit uncertain

I grew up watching the hit series *ER* on television. I was consistently and deeply impressed by George Clooney, in particular, striding forth with immediate and accurate diagnoses, saving lives with every breath taken by his stethoscope-clad chest.

I've been disenchanted – and not just because of Clooney's later treacherous liaison with Nestlé. I imagined that, just as in *ER*, medicine would be a place of dynamic decisions, distinct results and immediate action. I thought that we would ask what was wrong, take blood, X-rays, read the results and start the treatment. A medical degree would launch me forth with just the same ability; I would be just as capable as Clooney, slicing through with precise medical knowledge, kept up to date with every journal my post box could throw at me. How naïve, how wrong I was.

Every couple of weeks, as a junior doctor, I would be required to attend pathology meetings. This was all about the 'tissue diagnosis'. My responsibility was to fetch the notes, put them in order, introduce the clinical history ('Mrs Smith, a 72-year-old retired teacher who has had deteriorating renal function over the past year and presented with nephrotic syndrome two weeks ago') and then write down the conclusions of the discussions about Mrs Smith's kidney biopsy. Attending the meeting would be the surgeons and physicians. Playing God were the pathologists, who came with slides of those tissue samples and who were going to tell us what they meant. The slides, which were in whorls of pink and blue, were transmitted via projector to a white screen in front, on which we all held a concentrated gaze. And what did those pathologists say?

Before I tell you that, I tell you this. Biopsies are meant to be the bee's knees when it comes to diagnosis. They are the definitive answer. If you don't know what a lump is or what is happening in a liver or a kidney, then going to great lengths to obtain a little bit of that tissue, then preparing a sample to examine under the microscope, is what you are to do next.

Except the vocabulary of the pathologists didn't consist of words like 'definite', 'absolutely' or 'clearly'. What I remember most about those meetings is the pathologists questioning the physicians and the surgeons, wanting more details about when symptoms came, what happened next and what the other test results were. They talked about 'probably' and 'I think' and 'more than likely'. They often came back with several more ideas to explore and recommendations for more avenues of diagnosis. Pathology, that specialist field, described as the 'gold standard' of diagnosis,[1] was not capable of producing clear answers to everything. Pathologists needed more information – and were prepared to change a diagnosis according to what new information was shared by the clinicians looking after the patient.

Those valiantly obtained tissue slides were not the oracle. There was no 'god'.

Evidence demonstrates this uncertainty in pathological diagnosis time and again. A series of sarcomas, a type of bone tumour, were examined by three pathologists after the tissue samples had been assessed by pathology and a diagnosis given. Of the 216 patients, the pathologists agreed about the diagnosis 66% of the time. Many of these disagreements were about the exact type of tumour, but in 6% of patients, the diagnosis of cancer was disputed.[2] In a series of 49 ovarian tumours, when pathologists looked only at the tissue, having no information about the patient, there was absolute agreement about the diagnosis in 75% of patients. The rest were disputed, mainly about whether this was cancer or not.[3] Or take another study, this time looking at expert pathologists' diagnosis of skin cancer, where they were asked to categorise a slide tissue sample into either malignant, benign or indeterminate. In 38% of slides there were at least two disagreements between the experts; in these cases they were unable to agree whether a tissue sample diagnosed a cancer or not.[4]

This is rather important. A diagnosis of cancer may result in major surgery, chemotherapy and radiotherapy, all of which come with the chance of complications or damage. It may come with work, family, insurance and financial implications. And it all may be unnecessary if your diagnosis is wrong to start with.

I realise this may sound heretical. It isn't: here I will defend pathologists. If you have ever seen a tissue slide, stained with dye, you will know that it contains a barrage of shapes and colours. Pathology is partly about pattern recognition but it is also about quantities of cells, the position of cells and their shape. There is no such thing as an easily recognisable pattern that is repeated as faithfully as that on a Fair Isle jumper. The same pattern – say the cellular changes that happen in inflammation – can be caused by many different things. Pathologists are not stupid, either. They have a full medical training of five years followed by another five years of postgraduate training and exams, which are well known to be tough.

There could be a couple of explanations here. Pathologists may not be that good at their job. Or could it be that there is an inherent uncertainty to diagnosis, which it is *not possible* to reduce to zero?

For example, the *Journal of the American Medical Association* published an article about how to distinguish between a benign skin mole and a malignant melanoma. It listed the things to look out for (irregular colour, itch, bleeding, asymmetry) detailing the kinds of things that doctors should use to get to the truth, as demonstrated with a tissue biopsy. Biopsy, they concluded, was the answer. But a couple of doctors replied, with a disquieting candour:

> 'Their discussion demonstrates that they fully realise the limitations of the clinical examination, but they fail to acknowledge that the 'gold standard' of their study, microscopic examination of the biopsy specimen, has similar limitations. Without the certainty of a true gold standard of biological behaviour, all their inferences are suspect.'[5]

I'm afraid it's true: we are all, doctors and patients alike, guddling around in uncertainty, and this same uncertainty is the very nature of diagnosis – just as it is of screening. Sure, we can hone the odds a bit, we can gather more information to help us handle the slippery nature of our clinical dealings, but the ultimate conclusion is just the same. We can be as sure as we can possibly be that we are right – and later, shown to be wrong.

A study of almost 3,000 patients with lymphoma, a cancer of the immune system, in Canada suggested that around 15% had a questionable diagnosis with a result of substantial doctor-mediated harm in two-thirds of these.[6]

We may like to pretend that we have all the answers, or, at least, most of them. It's also tempting to think that if a doctor is kind, intelligent, hard working and up to date, then he or she will have all the answers. It may also be tempting to think that doctors are pathetic incompetents who think they know all the answers and only know a little. The truth, I think, is in between. Even doctors who are as angelically close to earthy perfection as possible are still going to get things wrong – simply because it is not possible to always get things right.

Bayes, balance and humanism

The relevance of an 18th-century minister and amateur mathematician to the demands of modern medicine may not be immediately apparent. Yet the Reverend Thomas Bayes understood something about complex decision making and uncertainty that many observers and practitioners of medicine do not.

It is essentially this: a small piece of information can transform the direction of travel of medical decision making. Let's take Mr Brown.

Mr Brown is breathless. Not very much, he says, just a bit, when walking uphill or for long distances. He's aged 65. He's not had any serious medical problems before. He stopped smoking when he was 30. He's just retired as a senior civil servant.

This is typical general practice. A problem with potentially dozens of causes. Let's see: Mr Brown could have a lung tumour, bronchitis, pneumonia, or fibrosis of the lungs (causing his lungs to be inefficient, unable to transfer oxygen-rich air into the bloodstream). He might have asthma, anaemia (insufficient red blood cells to transport enough oxygen through the blood) – or he could be simply overweight. His heart may not be pumping properly, because of a weakness in the cardiac muscle, or the blood vessels supplying that cardiac muscle (such as angina) or a valve problem in the heart preventing the blood leaving at the correct time. The heart may be beating erratically. There may be a blood clot, or multiple blood clots, on the lung. The breathlessness may be due to anxiety or panic attacks. I could go on but you get the idea. One symptom can have many causes.

To try to sort this out, the first thing to do is take a good history. If Mr Brown tells me that, since retiring, he has been feeling very low, purposeless and depressed, I will listen carefully for any hints that going out may be making him feel anxious and panicky. As well as listening to his story, I need to ask him questions: how is his sleep? (Sleep is often disturbed in anxiety conditions). Has he felt that life may not be worth living? Yes, he says, he is actually tormented by thoughts of suicide. He panics when his phone rings because then he will have to speak to someone. He is feeling desperately low. He may tell me that he is also very anxious because he is worried about the cause of his breathlessness. Last night he woke up with a heaviness over his chest. He woke up with it. Yes, the pain went down his left arm...

...and that is what makes my fingertips tap out 999, right away. That little bit of information – waking up with chest pain – trumps everything else. No matter what else he says – that yes, it could be depression and anxiety or even bronchitis because he has started smoking again, or perhaps asthma because it seems worse when he walks by cherry blossom trees – it doesn't matter. He's had chest pain so bad it woke him up. This chest pain fits the pattern for heart disease. He may have had a heart attack, or be having one now. If I don't diagnose anaemia or panic attacks immediately, it doesn't matter as much; the diagnosis that can't wait is that of a heart attack. That's the one that is immediately life threatening if I get it wrong.

Mr Brown could certainly get chest pain as part of an anxiety syndrome. But waking up with chest pain isn't common. I can't reasonably put this down to an acute anxiety attack – I need to exclude a dangerous cardiac cause.

This small piece of information about chest pain changes the direction of travel. It's an example of Bayes' theorem in action.

Thomas Bayes' theorem was that 'the pre-test odds of a hypothesis being true multiplied by the rate of new evidence generates post-test odds of the hypothesis being true.'[7] The hypothesis relates to what you think is wrong with the patient. The evidence is that of a symptom, or a blood test.

The way you interpret the meaning of a test depends on the knowledge you already have. In many ways the workings are the same as those discussed in Part One when we looked at the numbers behind screening tests. If a patient is pretty likely to have a condition, but a test for that condition is negative, it may be more likely that the result is a false negative not a true negative. So if I think my patient has had a heart attack, I shouldn't let a normal heart tracing, an ECG, stop me phoning an ambulance. ECGs can sometimes be normal in the early stages of a heart attack. But in medicine, information rarely appears in isolation.

Bayes' genius was to realise that this additive information can change the direction of travel rapidly. One small bit of highly relevant information can turn the tables upside down.

Here is an example from a *BMJ* paper I'm very fond of, entitled 'Why clinicians are natural Bayesians'.[7]

Doctor: How long have you had a fever?

Patient: Three days.

(Doctor thinks: sounds like an acute infection, probably a cold).

Doctor: Where have you been recently?

Patient: Libreville, in Gabon.

(Doctor thinks: well now, this might be a tropical infection, perhaps malaria, typhoid, tuberculosis, some kind of parasite. . ..or possibly one of those esoteric viruses we learned about at medical school).

Doctor: What did you do there?

Patient: I was part of a compassionate relief team helping rural villagers, many of whom were dying with bleeding gums, high fever, cough and skin rash.

(Doctor thinks: hmmm, esoteric virus quite plausible).

Doctor: Do you have those symptoms too?

Patient: Yes, my gums bleed when I brush, I have a painful skin rash, and I'm coughing blood (cough, cough).

(Doctor thinks: nasty esoteric virus very likely. Need to get this patient isolated and call Centers for Disease Control and Prevention, and Department of Homeland Security. Have I just been exposed to Ebola virus?).

The authors point out that the patient's symptoms of gum bleeding and skin rash are not specific to Ebola virus – there are hundreds of causes of these from dental infection to vitamin C deficiency – but because the patient has given the information suggesting that he is at high risk of Ebola virus, he is treated differently. Automatically, these become less likely to be symptoms of gum disease or heat rash and more likely to be those of a deadly virus.

Medical students learn how to take a history from a patient by first enquiring about the presenting complaint. This is the one

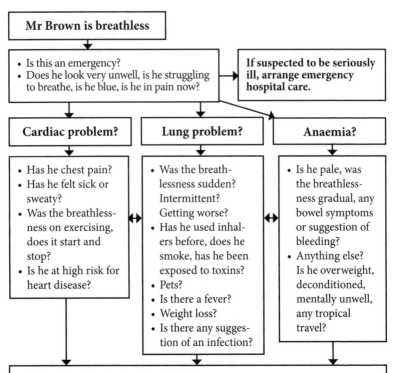

Mr Brown is breathless

- Is this an emergency?
- Does he look very unwell, is he struggling to breathe, is he blue, is he in pain now?

If suspected to be seriously ill, arrange emergency hospital care.

Cardiac problem?

- Has he chest pain?
- Has he felt sick or sweaty?
- Was the breathlessness on exercising, does it start and stop?
- Is he at high risk for heart disease?

Lung problem?

- Was the breathlessness sudden? Intermittent? Getting worse?
- Has he used inhalers before, does he smoke, has he been exposed to toxins?
- Pets?
- Is there a fever?
- Weight loss?
- Is there any suggestion of an infection?

Anaemia?

- Is he pale, was the breathlessness gradual, any bowel symptoms or suggestion of bleeding?
- Anything else? Is he overweight, deconditioned, mentally unwell, any tropical travel?

- What does examination show?
- Is he breathing fast or slow? Are his lips blue?
- Is he sweaty, or pale?
- What's his pulse, in rhythm and rate, and his blood pressure?
- What do his heart and lungs sound like, and does his abdomen feel normal?
- Is there a cough? Is it characteristic of any particular disease? What's his peak flow (a measure of how quickly air can be blown through a tube)?
- Is there ankle swelling ?
- Any lymph node enlargement?
- Any evidence of weight loss, or fever?

- Does this need tests? How quickly?
- Should he be admitted into hospital, or should out-patient tests be done?
- Do we need an ECG of the heart, a chest X-ray, breathing tests, a treadmill cardiac test?
- Should we check bloods for blood count, and for markers of infection, or send a sputum sample?
- Are we very suspicious of a lung disorder and do we need to consider further tests even if the chest x-ray is normal?

Making a diagnosis.

that has caused you to be a patient today. Then you are asked about your history of medical problems and your family medical problems. Then there is time to ask about employment, housing, if you smoke, how much you drink, if you have dependants or someone to look after you, and, if relevant, where your toilet is. Then there is 'systematic enquiry'. Your respiratory system: are you breathless, do you wheeze, do you have a cough? Your urinary system; any pain when you pee, any blood, going more often than usual? And so on, through your neurological, gastroenterological, dermatological, rheumatological and vascular systems until a comprehensive total of your symptoms – a properly holistic history – is recorded.

This takes time. The more experienced the doctor, the more he or she will ask questions to exclude or include a 'differential diagnosis' – that honing down of possibilities into a more distinct hypothesis about what is wrong with you. Bayes' theorem is a good description of how medicine is practised. Diagnosis is instantly responsive, malleable and intelligent to new information.

Binary medicine

Bayesian thinking is remote to the modern method of diagnosis: the protocol. It's a bit like a flowchart, with questions leading to yes/no answers, which then lead on to further yes/no answers and finally an action. Protocols were rare when I was a student but now I have a special shelf just to deal with their bulky forms when they arrive in my office. Protocols are closely related to guidelines, which are not usually to do with diagnosis but treatment. Guidelines are issued by everyone from the Royal Medical Colleges to the Department of Health to NICE and every local service your NHS has to offer. I have hundreds of glossy guidelines, their weight creating saggy curves in the shelves that struggle to contain them.

The idea has always been that guidelines can be used to reduce variation and increase uniformity in how healthcare is used.

'Humans have only a limited ability to incorporate information in decision making. In certain situations, the mismatch between this limitation and the availability of extensive information contributes to the varying performance and high error rate of clinical decision makers. Variation in clinical practice is due in part to clinicians' poor compliance with guidelines and recommended therapies. The use of decision-support tools is a response to both the information revolution and poor compliance.'[8]

This was written in a mainstream US medical journal, the *Annals of Medicine*, in 2000. It is typical of the view that more standardisation means better practice. Clinicians are depicted as outlaws, wilfully ignoring the best treatment for their patients. Guidelines are seen as the graceful saviour, pointing out the correct path and the most effective intervention. A systematic review of computerised 'clinical decision support systems [CDSSs]' – online versions of protocols – was published in the *Journal of the American Medical Association* in 2005, and concluded that:

'There is currently widespread enthusiasm for introducing electronic medical records, computerised physician order entry systems, and CDSSs into hospitals and outpatient settings. In other commercial, industrial and scientific spheres of activity, computers have become ubiquitous and have improved safety, productivity, and timeliness. Given this progress, computerisation of the health care environment should offer tremendous benefits. However, uptake has been slow, and multiple challenges have arisen at every phase of software development, testing, and implementation. The progress of CDSSs have mirrored these trends. . . These evaluations have shown that many CDSSs have improved practitioner performance.'[9]

Now, true, I've spent a good part of this book describing how doctors are bad at thinking about evidence and have a worrying tendency to do things according to their opinion, not the evidence. I truly believe that without acting on the evidence it's easy to harm, maim or kill patients, even when you think you are doing good.

So aren't guidelines the solution to this problem? Don't good guidelines, based on quality evidence, impart scientific credentials to harried clinicians and not-quite-up-to-date doctors, and arm patients with a decent idea of what good practice is?

I wouldn't disagree that some guidelines are capable of doing some good. Of larger concern, though, is the way in which protocols and guidelines are kicking their spiky heels into the very core of medicine, overturning the evolved Bayesian nature of medical practice.

Protocols are loved by managers and politicians because they are easy to follow. (Note: I haven't said anything about their accuracy or flexibility.) The easier a protocol is to follow, the less training a person needs to apply it; it seems simple, straightforward and immediately clear. It's quite easy to follow a computer programme that gives you nice choices: yes or no. However, problems begin if the answer to the question: 'Do you have chest pain?' is not 'yes' or 'no' but 'well maybe', or 'I don't think so', or 'actually, I had some chest pain last week'. Making sure everyone gets a high standard of healthcare is a good thing. But trying to shoehorn patients into rigid boxes is not helpful.

In reality, variability in medical practice is sometimes good. What if you don't just send women breast screening appointments but offer them discussions about whether or not they wish to have breast screening? Uptake of breast screening may fall. Some people would argue that this is a harmful situation; I would suggest that it's unethical to offer people anything other than good information to make decisions and to rely on their choice, not mine, on whether or not to have it. What about statin prescribing? Supposing my patients have far fewer statins prescribed to them than other general practices nearby. The easiest conclusion would be that I have veered off protocol and that I am not applying the guidelines as they should be applied to my patients. But perhaps I am offering my patients evidence with which to make the choice themselves, and not automatically hitting the 'prescribe' button every time a high cholesterol rears into view.

The conclusion that variability is bad is distant from the much simpler observation that patients are all different. Patients want different things. Some people will do anything to avoid a surgical operation. Others don't mind about that but really don't want to take pills. Some will find it easy to lose weight to control blood pressure. Other people want to do everything they possibly can to avoid a complication, even if they have substantial side-effects from the tablets required.

8

The snowballing of protocols

Protocols pride themselves on the distillation of evidence such that they are easy to follow; this, in the view of some, makes them suitable to be used by people with minimal training. The research becomes a simple flowchart fitting nicely onto a notice board or desk, abbreviating multiple studies into quick decisions. Yet there is seldom room for 'perhaps', or to reflect on any uncertainties thrown up by the studies making recommendations.

All the evidence we have – everything on which we base our protocols and guidelines – retains an inherent uncertainty. The Scottish Intercollegiate Guidelines Network (SIGN) grades evidence by its quality. It tags each of the individual statements in its guidelines with an indication of how much reliability can be attached to it.

So for example, the 'top quality' mark goes to high-quality meta-analyses, systematic reviews and randomised controlled trials with a low risk of bias. These are the most reliable forms of science. It is only this level of evidence that will result in what SIGN calls a 'grade A' recommendation, which is the highest type of endorsement.

And right enough, languishing at the bottom of the evidence hierarchy we find 'expert opinion', which can only be counted towards a 'grade D' recommendation.

I rather like the SIGN way of doing things because it makes

it clear that applying evidence is all at least a little bit uncertain, with some things being rather less uncertain than others. But do the people using guidelines remember this and adapt what they are doing accordingly?

How would we know? We would need evidence of clinical judgments that are capable of changing in the light of what patients tell us, both about what has happened to them and about their preferences for what happens next.

The unquestioning use of protocols may not even help patients at all.

24/7 triage

NHS Direct, launched in 1998, was the first big official telephone advice line for patients in urgent need of help. Most out-of-hours services until then had been staffed by local GPs, who would often work in co-operative groups to answer phones, offer appointments to patients who were able to travel to them, and visit those who weren't. Telephone triage – judging the relative urgency of each patient's call – had been an art practised by doctors and was learned by osmosis. An essential part of my GP training was to sit next to an experienced GP who was himself taking calls out of hours, then take the calls myself with the GP listening in, ready to intervene if I was getting it wrong. This process took place for six hours, at least once a week, for a year. And remember, this was as part of GP training, after five years at medical school and a further two years of hospital jobs. GPs had been doing this kind of work as a natural progression, switching between triage, seeing patients who came in, or doing home visits as needed. These doctors were using their medical knowledge to deal with any problem presented to them. There was no single guideline they referred to.

When NHS Direct was rolled out, the idea was that it would be staffed by nurses, with an average of four weeks' induction training.[1] A first analysis of how well NHS Direct was working was performed by the Medical Care Research Unit of Sheffield

University for the Department of Health in 1998.[2] There was, though, no clear evaluation of how accurate, or how efficient, the telephone advice was. The 'critical event monitoring' done was initially by 'surveillance of local press for all reports relating to NHS Direct', then by 'liaison with coroners' and finally by 'identification of hospital admissions/A&E attendances with index conditions (such as meningitis, suicide and parasuicide, and non-accidental injury) and ascertainment of whether a call to NHS Direct preceded the admission/attendance'.

Trusting in the quality of the local press is not a reliable way to gather evidence of harm; we need proper, detailed, controlled studies to do that. Instead, the evidence for the effectiveness of NHS Direct was gathered post-hoc, after the political decision had been made to implement it. Evidence was not leading practice, politics were. Assessments of the service initially focused on patient 'satisfaction' but precious little attention was paid to clinical accuracy. Is this good enough?

What protocols and guidelines mean for patients

The truth is that we don't know a lot about how good protocol-based advice lines are. Instead of being able to deal with any problem in any individual situation, and adjusting medical care to take account of evidence and patient preference, only one size of protocol is available. Patients may be fortunate enough to find an operator with skill who can override a protocol if necessary – or they may not.

Here is an example of the kind of thinking that results from guidelines. NHS guidelines state that cervical smears should be performed three-yearly on women over the age of 25. What happens if a woman visits her GP with an unrelated matter? Well, 'guidelines' state that this woman is at risk of cervical cancer. An element of GPs' pay depends on how many of the eligible women on their practice list have smears. Here's what one GP, herself a trainer of GPs, thinks should happen. This is an extract from a 'How to' series in a popular GP magazine.

'Mrs Brown has come today with a cough. You notice from her records that she has not had a smear for 10 years. . .'

Why hasn't Mrs Brown had a smear?

She may have slipped through the net . . . She may think that she must be all right because she has no symptoms, that a single smear is sufficient, or that smears only detect cancer and are therefore pointless. Monogamous and currently celibate women often mistakenly believe they are not at risk.

However, she may be deliberately avoiding smears through embarrassment, because she has symptoms that she secretly worries are cancer or sexually transmitted, has vaginal dryness, or because she found her last smear upsetting (women still occasionally report lack of privacy or a chaperone, or that their examination was rough or painful). Sensitive questioning may allow her to reveal the real reason without feeling embarrassed or ignorant . . .

What if Mrs Brown still refuses?

All women should be offered advice about risk factors for cervical cancer as well as contraception where appropriate, and sexually transmitted diseases. This can be done as part of health promotion, a well-woman service, or opportunistically. Some women get irate if they are asked repeatedly. It is not ethical either to badger Mrs Brown or to remove her from the list for the sake of reaching cytology targets.

Mrs Brown should be told that she can change her mind, and may well do so, having thought about it or discussed it with relatives or friends. Her records should show that she has been offered both a smear and relevant advice.[4]

Now all those things might be true. Perhaps Mrs Brown is secretly yearning for a cervical smear and desperate for her doctor to notice that she is due one. You'll notice that Mrs Brown is not to be forcibly put on the treatment table, legs in stirrups and smeared – not quite. However, there is no room – absolutely no credence given – to the idea that Mrs Brown might just be a competent adult who has weighed up the pros and cons of screening and thought: I don't want this smear, thank you. One is not allowed to be a person who 'chooses not to have' or to 'decline', one is only allowed to be a 'refuser'. Language, here, is especially important. To decline speaks of one who has decided; to refuse speaks of belligerent anti-socialism. There is just a nod to non-enforcement with the note that she should not be 'badgered' but that's it.[5]

The fact that there is no reasonable alternative route avoiding smears is a direct result of the way in which healthcare is generically provided. There is no crucial assessment, right at the start, of whether the person wishes to embark on this 'protocol' and become a patient. No other route is offered. Once you are on that route, it is incredibly hard to get off it again. As in the discussion above, the main issue addressed is *how* to get that woman to have her smear, not *if* she wants it done in the first place.

There is not a 'quick exit' with a protocol – you have to keep going. You can't ditch the whole lot, Bayesian style (ah – the thinking, Bayesian-style doctor notes – this woman has written to us and told us she doesn't want a smear, she found it distressing, and wrote to tell us so), and get quickly to the right destination.

Money and protocols

Protocols are not the only barrier towards individualised care. The intrinsic workings of the NHS provide plenty of bias towards placing people automatically on protocols. It's all about money.

As hinted at by the cervical smear story above, doctors are routinely rewarded – or, one could say, penalised – depending on how many boxes they are able to tick when it comes to services delivered. Family doctors are not employed directly by the NHS. Instead, ordinary GP surgeries contract to the NHS for delivering services. There are a few exceptions, for example, health centres owned and run by local government (usually by the local Primary Care Trust.) Such centres often directly employ doctors and nurses to work in a built-for-purpose office but they are the exceptions.

As contractors to the NHS, GPs' money follows specific activities. There are hundreds of categories for payment, from childhood vaccinations, to the number of 'temporary residents' seen, to contraception offered and, of course, cervical screening. Each 'activity' attracts a specific computer code, which is used to notify the Health Board or PCT that payment is due. The income to a general practice is made up of a myriad of little fees that have to be duly noted, added and claimed.

There are several types of services that practices get paid for. Core services are those that every practice has to provide and are covered under the Global Sum,[5] the practice's share of the basic amount allocated by the government for general medical services. The other types of payments fall into two main groups: the first is enhanced services, covering things like minor surgery and monitoring of patients taking the blood thinning drug warfarin. The second are payments under the Quality and Outcomes Framework (QOF).

The QOF was the result of negotiations between the trade union, the British Medical Association and the government in 2004. For example, injections into knees or shoulders for joint pain, done as part of a minor surgery service, attract about £40 each. Flu vaccinations pay £6.80 each.

The QOF is rather more involved. GPs are incentivised into reaching a variety of 'indicators'. So, if patients with heart disease are on the approved list of medications and have low cholesterols, the doctor gets points. If the doctor shows that these patients have been told to stop smoking and be a healthy weight, there are more points. Points mean cash.

There is a reasonable argument for paying doctors in this way. It goes like this: we need to be sure we are efficient. We should only pay for what we know to be effective medical care. We have evidence that suggests that stopping smoking, low cholesterol and blood pressure, and aspirin all reduce mortality after a heart attack. Therefore, we should base doctors' pay on their ability to provide such evidence-based services.

There is truth in there. Evidence matters. As we've said, doing things just because you think it's a nice idea is not compatible with good medical care. We need evidence and we should use it.

But the problem is that each one of these GP contract deals is really a concentrate of protocol. Heart attack? Statin, aspirin, ace inhibitor, beta blocker, flu vaccination. That's all the contract is really concerned with. As a patient, that's what you are reduced to.

There is an association between chronic ill health and depression. So the latest version of the QOF (it's reviewed annually, when more tick boxes are inserted) has two further questions: During the last month, have you often been bothered by feeling down, depressed or hopeless? and: During the last month, have you often been bothered by having little interest or pleasure in doing things?

The instigators of these little questions say that it's a good thing. Depression is common, they say, especially in people who have had a heart attack or stroke. So let's incentivise doctors to spot it; let's pay them to do so.

These questions are followed by a questionnaire asking about mood, sleep, and anxiety levels. To score full points, GPs must perform the same questionnaire a month after the initial one.

There are two massive problems with this incentive scheme: context and screening. The 'two questions' are not designed to diagnose depression, but to screen for it. They are not diagnostic tests.

Depression by numbers

Depression is, truly, a miserable affliction: I have encountered many people who have had both depression and unpleasant treatment for medical conditions and who will say the depression was easily worse. What follows does not denigrate this illness.

The problem for screeners is that not all low mood is depression. Questionnaires, when done as a reflex adherence to protocol, do not account for the circumstances people find themselves in. Life is not a straight emotional arrow. Our mood can sink when we are faced with bad news, an undesirable change in our circumstances, even just a stretch of jet lag-broken sleep. Normal people have moods that change according to what is happening to them. An enormous part of literature, art and music over the past few thousand years has been an attempt to understand and to share what life means through shared emotions.

The advent of the protocol-based questionnaire removes all context from assessing patients' mental states. From the beginning, there is no option for patients to say that they are distressed because their dog has died or they are feeling awful because they have flu. Instead, the questionnaire is administered, high levels of distress recorded and then the doctor or nurse deals with the result. Normal discourse between doctor and patient is relegated to second place behind the paperwork. The questionnaire-based screening for depression is capable of removing human understanding from the encounter between doctor or nurse and patient.

It's known that in some surveys, up to 95% of people, if asked, will admit to feeling low on a regular basis.[6] And it is also clear that most people are not incapacitated by 'depression' as diagnosed by such questionnaires. Indeed, true depression is relatively rare. When the very first antidepressant was developed in 1959, the manufacturers were disinclined to market it to doctors since the pharmaceutical company thought depression was an uncommon disorder and they were not likely to recoup the costs.[7]

All change. More than 40 million prescriptions for antidepressants – that's *forty million* – were written in the UK in 2010.[8] The question now becomes: how likely is the routine use of depression screening questionnaires to help patients? And how much harm does their use cause?

Indeed, before the instigation of the QOF, it was well known that screening for depression generally resulted in picking up low mood because of life events, and wasn't terribly helpful in finding new depression cases. In one study, researchers found that patients scoring high on questionnaires turned out not to be depressed when they interviewed them.[9] The ongoing problem has been this misunderstood differentiation. Studies that look at levels of distress tend to find lots of unhappiness, and conclude that depression is therefore underdiagnosed. Search for 'depression' and 'underdiagnosed' on any medical search engine, and there are hundreds of papers supporting that view.

There is a problem with this outlook. Surveys collect a snapshot, data taken at a single point in time. This is contrary to the usual way patients and doctors interact. So, patients who have a diagnosis of heart disease are the kind of patients who are regular attenders at the surgery, returning to have blood pressure checked or blood tests done, and who may well have other conditions too. Real life medicine is not a 'point in time', paper-based exercise. It is a relationship flowing over months and years.

And indeed, other studies have shown that most true cases of depression found at these 'point in time' studies have a habit of finding their way in the future to appropriate diagnosis and treatment anyway.[10]

So how accurate are the questionnaires? The ideal questionnaire with no false positive or negative results does not exist. One commonly used questionnaire, the PHQ (Patient Health Questionnaire), has been noted to be truly correct for depression only around half the time. The bottom line is this: 'good sensitivity but poor specificity'. Only between 30% and 60% of the time does a positive questionnaire screening score mean that the person really is depressed.[11,12]

Yet one of these studies concludes that the survey can be a 'reliable and valid measure of depression severity.' This is quite a jump, considering that the authors have just told us that their tool will get it wrong the majority of the time.

More, there is evidence that the different questionnaires that are still clinically validated and used by GPs for the purposes of cash by QOF are not themselves comparable – meaning that depression of different severity could be diagnosed in the same person with the same set of symptoms, just by the use of different questions.[13]

And here is the crunch point. Despite all the bits of paper flying around and patients being asked to tick boxes and practice staff being asked to type them into computers, this may all be a wasteful distraction. Doctors don't find them useful. Instead, they listen to their patients, ask them how life is, and try to put everything back in context. If the questionnaires were all that mattered, and the protocols for treating depression from NICE were followed to the letter, then three-quarters of people scoring as depressed would be started on antidepressants. But in practice, far fewer actually do end up on medication.[14]

So does depression by numbers do any good? Or does our eagerness to hone general practice down to an 'evidence based' set of protocols and ticksheets create fundamental departures from what the patient might actually want to talk about?

9

Who decides what doctors do: pharma, politicians or patients?

Modern medicine has created skewed priorities. People are made into patients, caused by the indiscriminate culture of screening. The paradoxical problem is of not getting medical care when you are sick and need it. What happens in the consulting room is no longer a straightforward exchange between patient and doctor. Instead, all kinds of external influences impact on this private conversation.

At medical school, and then within my postgraduate training, I was taught a very important thing: find out why the patient has come to you. Let them talk. Try not to cut in. If you want to know the diagnosis, listen to the patient, for they are telling it to you.

There are many 'consultation models' to which young doctors are told to refer in order to improve their communication abilities. All make it clear that you will fail unless you find out why the patient is there.

Some of the wisest advice I was given was to try not to interrupt for at least the first minute (routine GP appointments are generally ten minutes long.) Under pressure, knowing that you are running late, it is easy for the doctor to want to take control of the consultation and sort out the problem – or at least, what the doctor thinks is the problem.

Doctors were taught to try to allow patients to dictate what happened in the consultation. If patients wanted advice about the matter of back pain, headache, a sore knee or anxiety, this is their prerogative. Doctors were there to address their patients' complaints. Sure, if the doctor noticed that a blood pressure was due to be taken or that a long-term prescription also needed to be discussed, it might be reasonable to raise this – but only after the patient has had the chance to talk.

I qualified in the mid-90s, and there has been a slow slide away from the precedence of the patient's concerns. Instead, the consultation has become populated with directions that originate outside what either the patient or the doctor might reasonably want to talk about.

The GP contract is full of such directions. As soon as I invite a patient to come in and have a seat, a yellow box will pop up on my computer screen reminding me to ask the patient whether he or she smokes and whether I can help with stopping. There are similar 'contract indicators' liable to jump up for attention whenever a tickbox has been left unfilled, demanding the doctor pay attention and fill them in while the patient is there.

Certainly, we know that smoking is bad for you,[1] that doctors can help 'prompt' people to stop smoking[2] and that when you stop smoking, you gain years of better quality of life.[3] But what we haven't researched with the same spirit is the effect on the consultation when the doctor's contract-related priorities take precedence over what the patient originally wanted to talk about.

I have no doubt damage occurs. One patient – let's call her Yvonne – is a woman who is very overweight, has low self-esteem and who had a difficult childhood. She would love to have some help with her migraines, and suffers from debilitating depression every few years. Six years ago a nurse told her, at one of the 'routine new patient checks' that the GP contract insists on, that she was dangerously overweight. When she went to see a doctor a few weeks later, trying to keep her head held high, her weight was the first thing he mentioned. She felt humiliated. She has never been back to the doctor since.

I can't quantify the harms that such protocols have done, because we haven't looked for them. We have simply assumed that because they are based on evidence and good intentions, that is sufficient.

I don't think that good intentions are good enough. And neither is the GP contract the only external influence that presses doctors into doing things that may not be helpful to patients.

Pharma, doctors and patients

The next time you are seated in your doctors' consulting room, take a look around. What kind of pen is she using? Are the boxes of tongue depressors in flashy packaging? Do the calendars on the wall have the small words 'A gift from. . .' at the bottom? What about the clock? Is there the name of a drug company in red letters in the middle? Do the toys in the toybox appear to have been gifted by a pharmaceutical company?

If the answer to these is 'yes', it doesn't necessarily mean that your doctor has gone over to the dark side. I've been criticising drug representatives for the past ten years, refusing to see the reps sent to the surgery, yet still I often struggle to find a pen that isn't emblazoned with a pharma logo. Pharmaceutical tat has a way of wriggling in. Unfortunately.

In 2004, an inquiry by the parliamentary health committee investigated the workings of the pharmaceutical industry in the UK. It concluded that:

'The influence of the pharmaceutical industry is such that it dominates clinical practice, to an extent that deprives it of independent and constructively critical feedback . . . It seems that intensive marketing has worked to persuade too many professionals that they can prescribe with impunity.'

The committee was

'dismayed to find that there is no register of interests to record gifts, hospitality or honoraria received by prescribers'.[4]

Indeed, free pens are the least of the problems. Drug reps are usually youngish, attractive men and women who are sent by their pharmaceutical company to 'educate' doctors and nurses about their products. These products are normally new, and expensive. I have sat politely through tedious explanations of how marvellous a drug is, accompanied by shiny graphs that lacked labels on their axis. Once, on questioning what the axes were meant to be, I was frowned at by a smartly dressed woman who informed me that I was the only doctor to ask such a thing, and she had spoken to some very senior people indeed. Some GPs have been 'gifted' branded stethoscopes, and the anointed few who allow regular visitations from reps get laser pointers, memory sticks, oodles of boxes of tissues and other assorted rubbish. Some reps would even swoop in with chocolates to pep you up as they talked you through the latest pharmacological breakthroughs.

The next step up for the eager doctor is the pharma-sponsored meeting. I (still) get a couple of invites a month, typically to a five star hotel, where I am promised a buffet and wine if I stay for a talk, delivered by a local 'expert' in whatever condition they are 'educating' you about. Attendees' names are discreetly taken and they will be called on in a week or two to ask how their prescribing is going.

Of course the 'expert' is paid, usually a few hundred pounds. The audience may be too: I was once offered £200 to attend one such 'educational' meeting. Once an 'expert' has been brought into the pharma fold, the world may be his oyster. If he continues to supply what the pharmaceutical company want to pay for, further assignments will follow. National meetings and then international meetings can follow, perhaps a research programme, to which funding comes easy. The resorts are always sunny and starry; life for the expert becomes easier.

This may be happening in your back garden, but it is not a cottage industry. In the US, there is one pharmaceutical representative for every six doctors. Up to $57 billion is spent per year on promotion of medicines, almost double that spent on pharmaceutical research.[5] Indeed, pharmaceutical companies can buy lists of what doctors individually prescribe and then target individual doctors whose prescribing patterns they want to 'improve'.

This is not just happening stateside. In the UK, similar systems were developed by IMS Health, a company that sells 'end to end solutions', saying:

'Brands must excel at launch, and continue to soar. IMS helps clients optimise their commercial resources and enhance global planning and implementation,' because 'we are the only company that tracks more than 70 percent of global pharmaceutical sales . . . we also capture data about more than 260 million anonymised patients worldwide, including their diagnosis and treatment.' IMS appreciates that 'clients require a clearer picture of market dynamics to better understand and anticipate opportunities'.[6]

Corporate gobbledegook. It may not be clear that this company obtains – legally – patient anonymised data about prescriptions, which are then sold to pharmaceutical companies in order for them to market their products more 'effectively' at doctors.

Let's leave aside who pays for this immense data trawl, reports, glossy brochures and marketing analysis (for in the UK, that would be the NHS, which funds the pharmaceutical industry by purchasing its products) and look at the morality of the situation. Doctors and patients should make decisions together about what prescription drugs to use and when. Is it right that this information can be passed to third parties – albeit with some details removed – for marketing purposes?[7]

The data can be sold on to companies who will target the doctors they can make gains on. These are the doctors who will be approached by pretty, well dressed reps, who just want a few minutes of their time and to gift them 'calendars, note pads, pens, watches, gym bags, hats, umbrellas, t-shirts, backpacks, calculators, paper clips, magnets'[8] . . . or just a few notebooks and ice scrapers for your car.

What trivial items! So it goes; many doctors think they can't be bought with this kind of trivia. They think that a box of tissues and a few post-it notes will make no difference to what they think or what they do. They truly believe that the grindings of the pharmaceutical industry, which is assiduously tracking their signatures on their prescription pads, flattering their busyness and understanding their pressures, have nothing to do with what they prescribe. Indeed research shows that health professionals 'believe that pharmaceutical representative interactions improve patient care, and that they can adequately evaluate and filter information presented to them'.[9] One doctor working in the pharmaceutical industry defends it, arguing that critics

'. . . fear that physicians are so weak and lacking in integrity that they would "sell their souls" for a pack of M+M candies and a few sandwiches and donuts . . . Physicians in hospitals should not be denied contact with sales representatives and the useful information they can impart just because of the unfounded fears of a few'.[10]

But in fact doctors can be bought with silly little gifts quite easily (and do we really think that organisations with such enormous PR departments and a keen eye on results don't notice this?) Doctors who make frequent contact with sales reps are more likely to prescribe more expensive products.[11] A review of more than 500 studies examining the relationship between doctors and reps concluded that 'the present extent of physician-industry interactions appears to affect prescribing and professional behaviour'.[12] It goes on to say that doctors 'believe that representatives provide accurate information about their drugs'. Many doctors say that they are sceptical about the claims that pharma makes but their behaviour when it comes to writing prescriptions is still affected. We may think we can act independently of what the rep tells us. But several tons of plastic pens and multiple research papers tell us the opposite. Whether doctors like it or not, they are influenced by the contacts they have with industry. This means undue influence in the consulting room; another problem for the patient who wants evidence-based, not advertising-hyped, healthcare. Good intentions, once again, are not enough.

Trusting what we're told

Most pharmaceutical companies take grave exception to the idea that we shouldn't trust them. Instead, they tend to mount a defence that sounds to my ears like an attack. In the fallout of the parliamentary inquiry, Vincent Lawton, president of the Association of the British Pharmaceutical Industry, decided that since there had been a decline in sales of pharmaceutical drugs that year, action was needed.

> '[He] hit out at the reluctance of GPs to switch to new life saving medicines when they are approved for use in the NHS. "At times, the conservatism of British doctors borders on Luddism," Mr Lawton said. He added that rules were needed to force doctors to prescribe new treatments at the earliest opportunity. "There should be an obligation for GPs to take up new drugs as soon as they are approved. Doctors' rewards should be linked to their prescription record."[13]

In his book *Drug Truths: Dispelling the Myths about Pharma R&D* John L LaMattina draws on his experience as former head of Pfizer Global Research and Development to tell us how fantastic he believes his industry is. He quotes a colleague: 'We like to say here at Pfizer that "the patient is waiting"'. He concludes his book 'It is time that people recognised the pharmaceutical industry for its contributions and support it in the quest to take health care to a higher level.'[14]

So what higher level is that? Should we enter into a happy-clappy world where we all trust pharmaceutical companies when they tell us (or should that be *instruct* us GPs) what to prescribe?

Of course not. And here is why I don't – and you shouldn't – trust pharmaceutical marketing.

The Seroquel problem

An advert in a medical journal (if you are in the US, you will have adverts for this drug in newspapers and internet search engines too) shows a woman, curled into a fetal position, dressed in grey, sitting on grey, with greyish light trickling into the room. This is a picture of abject misery and of absolute suffering. The flash of print on the right hand side suggests that quetiapine is an adjunct treatment for depression or schizophrenia and, sold under the brand name Seroquel, will be enough to restore her happiness.

As we've already seen, low mood is common, depression far less common. Manic depression, now called bipolar illness, is less common still: rather than have downturns in mood, the person is susceptible to both downturns and upturns. A manic episode (upturn) is just as dangerous, with the person perhaps believing he has special powers or is secretly very rich and powerful, and acting accordingly.

Seroquel was advertised not just for the relatively rare disorders of bipolar illness and schizophrenia, but also as an 'add on' treatment for depression. It is not an antidepressant, as such, but from the group of drugs known as antipsychotics. Bipolar illness, until then, had been treated with not just antidepressants but other mood stabilisers such as lithium, an old drug that works well but must be carefully monitored. There are other mood-stabilising drugs such as carbamazepine, which is also used to control epileptic seizures. But this was different: an antipsychotic for depression.

The definition of 'bipolar' has broadened over the past decade. Piggybacking on it is a new condition 'bipolar 2', a disorder with fewer upswings than bipolar 1. People with bipolar 2 do not become truly manic, and do not have episodes where they believe they have, for example, special powers.

Bipolar 2 has been responsible for a massive upsurge in psychiatric diagnoses. A US study found that 'visit rates' to a doctor for youths – those aged up to 19 years – with a diagnosis of bipolar disorder had increased from 25 per 100,000 in 1994/5, to 1,003 in 2002/3. In adults, there was also an increase over the same period: from 905 per 100,000 to 1,679.[15]

This could be explained by better diagnosis, better recognition, or a genuine increase in the number of people with bipolar illness. Or it could be that a drug was created, marketed and prescribed by doctors listening to pharma advice and making more bipolar 2 diagnoses. If that was the case, one would expect to find that many diagnoses of 'bipolar' would not stand up to scrutiny. That's certainly what was found by a US study. Here, the researchers reviewed 700 patients with a diagnosis of 'bipolar'. They found, through interviews with the patients and self-administered patient questionnaires, that fewer than half the patients with the diagnosis truly met the criteria for it. The other half had been overdiagnosed with the condition, meaning that they were likely to be getting just the side-effects from treatment, not any benefit.[16]

Indeed, by the end of the 90s, one-seventh of the turnover of AstraZeneca, worth more than US$31 billion globally, was due to Seroquel. It had become what is known in the industry as a 'blockbuster'. By February 2010, however, John Blenkinsopp, AstraZeneca's former UK director, was claiming that he had been pressurised to deny that Seroquel could cause weight gain despite data he had been given showing that it could.[17] Adverts from the company showed that it was being marketed as a drug with a 'favorable weight profile' (other antipsychotic drugs had a tendency to weight gain as an undesirable side-effect.) In 2009, AstraZeneca agreed to pay US$520 million in total to the US Attorney's Office in Philadelphia to resolve investigations related to sales and illegal marketing of the drug.[18] In August 2010, AstraZeneca found itself paying out US$198 million in personal injury claims to 17,500 people for causing weight gain and diabetes.[19]

A little blip? An unforeseen unluckiness? Hardly. Internal emails from AstraZeneca point towards concealment. 'The larger issue is how do we face the outside world when they begin to criticise us for suppressing data' wrote their publications manager in an email in 1999, concerned that data from their own clinical trials might at some time reach the public. An internal review of their work had shown that almost a fifth of patients gained more than 7% of their body weight when on Seroquel. Another internal email says: 'Thus far, we have buried trials 15, 31, 56 and are now considering COSTAR' (another trial comparing Seroquel to an older antipsychotic).[20] The work that didn't suit AstraZeneca was made to disappear. It was made invisible, not published in any journal or the results made available to any other researchers working in the area. These emails only surfaced when they were cited as part of the evidence required for the courts in the US.

Moreover, it is apparent that drug companies were making concerted efforts to 'educate' doctors about bipolar 2 and to get them prescribing more for it. The US government lawsuit that cost AstraZeneca so much money claimed that Seroquel was being marketed outside its licence for other conditions such as anxiety and insomnia, mild depression and post-traumatic stress disorder. Worse, they did not market the drug only to psychiatrists expected to see patients with major mental illness frequently, but to primary care and paediatric doctors who would not normally initiate this kind of drug.[18]

In summary, a drug was marketed for a diagnosis of bipolar 2 – a condition that many people, on further examination, didn't actually have. The drug was advertised as being weight-neutral, when in fact AstraZeneca knew it wasn't and sought to suppress that fact. The drug was advertised outside its licence and to doctors who wouldn't normally prescribe to people with severe mental illness.

The weight of the pharmaceutical industry can easily slip between doctors and patients. Should we really trust the drug companies to 'educate' our doctors into better prescribing?

Vioxx and trust

Arthritis can be a disabling, painful and progressive disease. People with arthritis usually need painkillers to enable a good quality of life but the painkillers that are particularly useful, anti-inflammatories such as aspirin and ibuprofen (NSAIDs), also have gastric side-effects. This can lead to stomach irritation, erosion of the stomach wall, and occasionally bleeding and ulcers. So, if a drug came along that had the helpful anti-inflammatory effect but was safer on the stomach and could prevent gastric bleeding, it would be impressive.

This combination of anti-inflammatory and low risk of stomach problems was promised in Vioxx, or rofecoxib, a type of NSAID called a COX II inhibitor. Cox II's were theoretically going to reduce gastric complications while still giving good NSAID-type pain relief. A large randomised controlled trial, the VIGOR study, published in the *New England Journal of Medicine* (*NEJM*) in 2000 suggested that Vioxx was indeed safer than other, older NSAIDs.[21]

And doctors got prescribing. By the end of the 1990s, more than 80 million people globally had been prescribed Vioxx.[22] In fact, the US Food and Drug Administration (FDA) had approved Vioxx in 1999, 18 months before the VIGOR results were published. However, after the *NEJM* published the VIGOR study, staff at the journal noticed that results about cardiovascular effects were different from data made public at the FDA.[23] It took six months for a meeting to discuss this with the FDA. The *NEJM* felt that there were more heart attacks than expected in the Vioxx-treated group, and it was necessary to investigate this further with a trial to examine whether Vioxx was the cause. In the meantime, promotion for Vioxx continued apace. Educational meetings for doctors were arranged by Merck, the manufacturer, to 'debunk' concerns about cardiovascular side-effects, alongside an annual US$100 million spend in direct to consumer advertising in the US. The company kept up the pressure to prescribe with press releases, such as one entitled 'Merck Reconfirms Favourable Cardiovascular Safety of Vioxx'.[24]

The investigation by the *NEJM* concerning the number of heart attacks concluded that some relevant data were missing. However, it also seemed that the data appeared too late to be included in the VIGOR paper. Doctors, meantime, continued to prescribe Vioxx. But in 2005, subpoenaed information obtained during Vioxx litigation revealed that at least two of the authors of the VIGOR trial had, in fact, been aware of heart attacks that didn't end up in the published paper. The *NEJM* concluded:

'We determined from a computer diskette that some of these data (on cardiovascular safety) were deleted from the VIGOR manuscript two days before it was initially submitted to the Journal on May 18, 2000.'[24]

So there were concerns about cardiovascular safety in 2000, which were covered up. It took five more years for another paper, the APPROVE study, to be published in the *NEJM*. This was designed to look not at cardiovascular safety but at how useful Vioxx was in preventing bowel polyps. The conclusion was that Vioxx was useful in preventing them – and that taking it also increased heart attack and stroke risk. The study was halted prematurely because of this extra cardiovascular risk.[25] On this basis, on the 30th September 2004, Merck withdrew Vioxx from sale worldwide.[26]

Worse again, the *Lancet* published a meta-analysis about the cardiovascular safety of Vioxx in 2004, examining all the evidence available before 2004. It concluded, somewhat damningly, that 'rofecoxib should have been withdrawn several years earlier'.[27] The evidence in trials already out there existed to show that Vioxx carried more cardiovascular risks but if anyone in authority had noticed, they had done nothing about it. The editor of the *Lancet* concluded in an editorial: 'Vioxx, Merck and the FDA acted out of ruthless, short sighted, and irresponsible self-interest.'[28]

Still want to trust pharma to tell doctors what to prescribe?

Suicide and paroxetine

Suicide is the worst outcome of depression and the one that psychiatrists want most to prevent. There is an odd paradox when doctors are treating depression: the most worrying time may not be when patients are at their worst, but when they are getting better. When patients are most unwell, they may be unable to commit suicide because they cannot plan their thoughts well enough to do so. Having a partially treated depression – well enough to make and act on plans but still feeling suicidally depressed – can mean that the first few weeks of treatment can lead to a 'successful' suicide.

Thus, the treatment of depression with medication may have different effects than those expected. Making sure that antidepressants really do reduce, rather than increase, suicidal behaviour is vital.

In 2004, the then New York Attorney General, Eliot Spitzer, filed a suit against manufacturer Glaxo SmithKline (GSK), accusing it of fraud for withholding clinical trial results on the antidepressant Paxil (paroxetine) in children and adolescents. At the time, sales reps were visiting doctors telling them about the 'REMARKABLE efficacy and safety in the treatment of adolescent depression' when, in fact, none of their own data could support this.[29] GSK agreed to online publication of its studies done on adolescents and children, which were then analysed together in a new review. This concluded, in 2005, that 'the data strongly suggest the use of SSRIs (of which paroxetine is one) is connected with an increased intensity of suicide attempts per year.'[30] In 2007, the FDA ruled that all antidepressant medication should 'include warnings about increased risks of suicidal thinking and behaviour' in adolescents and young adults.[31]

By 2009, GSK had paid US$1 billion in lawsuits over Paxil, or paroxetine. While it is tempting to assume that what happens in the US has little bearing on what happens in the UK, this is, again, not the case. It does not matter where a research study has been done when it comes to promoting the outcomes for prescribing in the UK. Paroxetine was being prescribed in the UK to children. 'By concealing critically important scientific studies on Paxil, GSK impaired doctors' ability to make the appropriate prescribing decision for their patients and may have jeopardised their health and safety,' said Spitzer.[32]

It's not illegal to conceal trial data in the UK. This means that you may decide, as a patient, to take part in a clinical trial. You may do very well with the treatment, or placebo, or you may not. You may have side-effects related to the treatment being tested. You may even have serious side-effects – or possibly die because of the treatment under test. Yet there is *nothing illegal* about those results being shredded.

In 2004, Iain Chalmers, a health services researcher and

editor of the James Lind Library, wrote to the *BMJ* stating the problem quite clearly: 'Biased under-reporting of clinical trials kills patients and wastes money.'[33]

As I write, almost a decade later, nothing much has changed. A few companies have pledged to make all their results available, but there is still no legal protection for patients.

And pharmaceutical firms dismiss doctors like me, who have learned a healthy scepticism about new and old drugs, as 'luddites'.

Herceptin, hype and heart failure

The ways pharmaceutical companies push their agenda between doctors and patients is insidious. Doctors may neither acknowledge its influence, nor even know that their knowledge about a pharmaceutical product is incomplete, because data are being withheld.

In the UK, we do not have direct industry to customer advertising. But there are other ways for pharmaceutical companies to interfere with the way patients make decisions about treatments. Barbara Clark is a British nurse who was diagnosed with breast cancer in March 2006. She writes in her book, *The Fight of My Life,* about finding out about the drug Herceptin from reports in the newspapers.

> 'Because it hadn't been approved by NICE, it would not be available on the NHS. "You should try to get it" he [her oncologist] had urged "because it could increase life expectancy by a few per cent". A few per cent? The newspaper report suggested Herceptin would increase chances of survival by 50 per cent or more. Inevitably, Dr Hassan wasn't available – he was in Miami at the Roche trials, listening to the reports. The news was out, but he hadn't flown home yet and wouldn't be back at his clinic until the end of May – that was four weeks away. I spoke to his secretary: "I've seen the results. I want this drug. No matter how much it costs, I want it. I'm going to get it somehow. Even if it means going to America..."

As soon as Dr Hassan returned to the country, he rang me. "You're absolutely right, the results are astounding. This is a wonder drug. But I do have to warn you that it is exceptionally expensive and it will not immediately become available on the NHS to you. There is no doubt that the trials are exceptional."[34]

Clark proceeded to raise thousands of pounds from the public to fund her treatment. She describes handing out leaflets for fundraising, and suffering the humiliation of people walking by who 'don't know you're trying to save your life'. Indeed, even broadsheet newspapers joined in the clamour, with the *Observer* newspaper declaring Herceptin, in an editorial, to be an 'Instant cure-all' and demanding that it did not go through time-consuming checks with NICE, as would normally happen, and was instead made available immediately.[35]

When the drug for use in early breast cancer was first introduced, the results were greeted with vocal enthusiasm – unusual for an academic meeting. 'Probably one of the only standing ovations I will witness in my career was when (it was) presented by Edward Romand at the annual meeting of the American Society of Clinical Oncology,' said one witness.[36] The *Journal of the National Cancer Institute*, under the headline 'Trastuzumab steals show,' quoted a senior medical researcher as saying 'I have never seen anything like this in 25 years of breast cancer research.'[37]

So what was the cause of all the applause? The trial data compared standard treatment of breast cancer with standard treatment plus Herceptin in women with breast cancer who also had the HER-2 genetic code positive on their cancer. The trial had a median follow-up of two years, and the 'end point' – the main investigation of the trial – was disease-free survival. At two years, there was a difference of 'disease-free survival' of 9%. If you didn't get Herceptin, the chances of survival were 77%. If you got Herceptin as part of the trial, your survival rate was 86%.[38]

Now sure, that is a difference, and a potentially important difference. But was it worthy of such enormous hype? Clearly, Herceptin was not an 'instant cure all' – the chances were in favour of surviving breast cancer whether or not you got the drug. The assessment of the newspaper read by Barbara Clark of an increase of survival by 50% does not hold up to scrutiny.

Further, Herceptin, like any drug, has side-effects. Ovations were reported to the worldwide media, but there was less attention paid to the cardiac side-effects of the drug. In fact, survival at three years with Herceptin was 94.3%, versus 91.7% without.[39] Despite this narrow difference, an editorial in the same issue of the *NEJM* confirmed the media's impression of the academic community's wonder: 'The results are simply stunning . . . On the basis of these results, our care of patients with HER2-positive breast cancer must change today.'[40] Just a couple of lines provide caution: 'An unexpected observation in these phase 3 trials was the development of congestive heart failure in 2 to 16 percent of the patients who were treated with trastuzumab and chemotherapy' and 'Because of the high risk of recurrence and death in HER2-positive breast cancer, a rate of congestive heart failure of no more than 4 percent above that without trastuzumab was considered acceptable.'

Something interesting is happening here. A significant side-effect – cardiac failure – is noted, and has a quantification of uncertain frequency. Doctors are deciding on a percentage of patients in whom it is 'acceptable' to cause heart failure in balancing the advantages of taking trastuzumab. We should not be naïve – balancing acts of this type happen every time a prescription is signed and we take tablets or have an operation. But the problem here is that the risk was assumed to be one worth taking. An uncertainty was being dismissed while pressure was added to rush Herceptin through the drug approval process. And were patients being misled? The official website for Herceptin, which is run by Genentech, a part of the Roche group, expresses the headline benefits of Herceptin in relative rather than absolute risk, which we have already seen to be misleading.[41] In Clark's book, she talks of a 'one in 200 risk of serious heart problems'. An analysis published in 2006, however, found cardiac side-effects in 28% of patients taking the drug over three years, which seemed to reverse in most when it was stopped.[42] There remains a lack of information about very long-term side-effects after using it.

The hype was down to the academics, then. Hardly pharma's fault, is it?

Let's go back and examine just how unbiased we think the Herceptin glee has been. The HERA trial was itself sponsored by Roche and of the 32 authors listed on the paper, 18 declared fees for consulting, lectures, or grants from pharmaceutical companies, and four were employed by Roche.[43] Dr Hortobagyi, who wrote the *NEJM* editorial declaring that the results were 'simply stunning' and signified 'maybe even a cure' for breast cancer, is an adviser to breastcancer.org. The latter has received a contribution of more than US$100,000 from Genentech, and been given the high financial donor status of 'visionary'.[44]

In many ways it isn't surprising – there are few major drug companies able to fund big trials. But it does mean that there is an interconnectedness that could colour perceptions. Researchers naturally want their trials to show positive conclusions. Not only do they want drugs they test to be successful, they may also need them to be. A researcher once told me: 'It is your job to bring money into the university. If you don't get grants, you can consider yourself fired.' Researchers need good working relationships with their funders in order to survive. But were the relationships the researchers had with pharma – consultancy, lecture fees, grants – causing a bias in how much enthusiasm was generated, and then transmitted to the public?[45]

What does this mean for patients, trying to make sense of the data and make good decisions about their care? Barbara Clark threw herself into campaigning for the drug for herself and others, taking part in a huge media crusade. Ten-year-old daughters of women with breast cancer were having their letters to MPs released to the press saying: 'We would like our mum to be here when we grow up.'[46]

Jane Keidan was another woman with breast cancer who had heard the media's rallying cries to Herceptin in 2005. 'I was HER-2 positive,' she said, 'meaning that I could benefit from Herceptin.' She wrote to everyone she could think of, pleading to be given the drug. Keidan was also a doctor. 'I was fortunate because then

I also started to discuss it with other oncologists, an immense privilege. Basically it became clear that there wasn't a definitive answer in my own individual case.' She told me:

> 'Some colleagues said that on balance they'd use it; some others said they wouldn't – but they all said that they didn't really know. In the end I spoke to my oncologist. He allowed me to reach my own decision. He supported me when I came to the conclusion that, because it was all finely balanced and the data from the trials were immature, and because there was evidence of side-effects of Herceptin, my decision was going to fall on the side of not having it.' [47]

But still, you may ask, where was the pharmaceutical company promotion of Herceptin? Surely they were not culpable for overinflating a product and for creating all this publicity for themselves? They didn't need to. They had the researchers – but they also had healthcare charities.

10

Charities and favourite diseases

As a medical student and then junior doctor, I had a happily innocent view on healthcare charities. Some wanted to speak to us or send us information about 'their' illness or disease. As a junior I was insulated against the media to a certain extent: too busy to read newspapers and, before the easiness of the internet, it wasn't until my GP training that I started to realise that it wasn't just pharmaceutical companies that wanted to take me to task on what I wasn't or was prescribing for patients.

Healthcare charities were not just the benign creators of coffee morning fundraisers and sympathy. No, they had firm opinions on what I was and wasn't good at, what I was and wasn't aware enough of, and what I should be saying, doing and prescribing. After five years at medical school and several more in various hospital jobs, the message that I was in dire need of straightening out was bewildering and unpleasant. This was the kind of thing I started to realise was directed at me.

'Awareness of the gravity of stroke in the UK is alarmingly low amongst both the general public and some health professionals according to a new survey released today by the Stroke Association' (2004).[1]

'Part of the problem is lack of awareness among GPs, says the charity.' (Patients Association, 2006.)[2]

'GP awareness of HIV is frequently found to be lacking.' (Terence Higgins Trust, 2010).[3]

'A lack of awareness of ovarian cancer symptoms among both women and health professionals can contribute to delays in diagnosis. . .' (Target Ovarian Cancer, 2011).[4]

'Despite the prevalence of arrhythmias, there is relatively little awareness and understanding of heart rhythm disorders amongst the public, patients and healthcare professionals.' (Written evidence to parliament from the Arrhythmia Alliance, 2010).[5]

Many healthcare charities queue up to offer instruction to doctors about how they should manage patients. Some want to campaign, challenge and lead the direction of research, government policy, or, indeed, what GPs and patients say to one another in consulting rooms.

One could easily conclude, from dedicated reading of the media's opinion of doctors, that we are feckless and ignorant creatures, requiring to be cajoled into work and given basic education at every opportunity. We should not be surprised, therefore, when decision making about what drugs the taxpayer should fund is the subject of campaigns by charities, such as the Breast Cancer Campaign. The charity won the 'Best in-house team' accolade in a PR award ceremony. Its role in the 'Herceptin affair' was 'an example of a highly effective, integrated and effective team that developed and maintained a high national profile over a relatively short space of time,' said the judges, giving the prize in 2006.[6]

Were breast cancer charities a fair and reliable source of information about Herceptin? When Jane Keidan heard about Herceptin, she went online to the Breast Cancer Care website where she signed up to their campaign to make Herceptin available to all HER-2 positive women. 'I simply could not understand from the data presented on the website and in the media why such an effective treatment should be denied to women,' she wrote.[7] Indeed, the major breast cancer charities in the UK welcomed Herceptin enthusiastically. The Breast Cancer Campaign did not raise concerns about side-effects or efficacy, but contented itself with the comment that:

> 'We must remember that there is still another key step that Herceptin has to go through, which is the NICE and the SMC (Scottish Medicines Consortium) approval process for the use of Herceptin by the NHS. Campaign hopes that NICE and the SMC will approve the use of Herceptin quickly and that the resources will be in place to ensure that when this happens, this treatment, which will benefit one in four breast cancer patients in the UK, will be available to all these patients regardless of where they live.'[8]

Putting this in persepective, one in four breast cancers are HER-2 positive and are then suitable for treatment with Herceptin. We know that an extra 2.6% of HER-2 positive women who use Herceptin will be alive because of it after three years; the vast majority would have been alive without Herceptin. So for every 200 women just diagnosed with breast cancer, Herceptin will be able to extend the life of, overall, one of them. This is important – but it is very different from the enormous enthusiasm with which the drug was launched.

There was no braking. Jane Keidan almost became a poster girl after tabloid newspapers contacted her for quotes. Other women did dress up in pink and allow themselves to be photographed, pleading for the drug. Breast cancer charities were prominent in the press, asking questions about when the drug would be approved by NICE and for widespread use. Another charity, CancerBacup, now part of Macmillan Cancer support, identified a 'dossier of delay', which it felt was preventing faster approval of the drug for use on the NHS. Internationally, there was much excitement. Breast Cancer Action Australia, which had previously made a young mother 'the face of the Herceptin campaign' in recurrent breast cancer, convened 'stakeholder' meetings and pushed for the drug's availability.[9]

Little attention had been paid to an editorial in the *Lancet* in November 2005, which called for caution. 'The excitement is premature,' it said:

'The studies so far reported represent interim efficiency analyses. As Victor Montori and colleagues advised in last week's *JAMA* (*Journal of the American Medical Association*), such analyses may 'show implausibly large treatment effects'. They recommend that 'clinicians should view the results of such trials with scepticism'. The two *NEJM* reports use different dosing regimens, making comparisons and conclusions additionally more difficult. It is especially hard to tease apart the results because one of the papers combines results from two trials sponsored by Genentech. . . The best that can be said about Herceptin's efficacy and safety for the treatment of early breast cancer is that the available evidence is insufficient to make reliable judgments. It is profoundly misleading to suggest, even rhetorically, that the published data may be indicative of a cure for breast cancer.'[10]

In other words, the trial data held uncertainties, hazards and concerns. Were these translated by breast cancer charities into good enough, balanced enough, sage enough advice for women in the throes of a new diagnosis of breast cancer and who needed information about their treatment? It is pertinent to note that in the UK, Breakthrough Breast Cancer, the Breast Cancer Campaign and Breast Cancer Care, all of whom campaigned vigorously for trastuzumab, have all received funding from the pharmaceutical industry.

In fact, only two breast cancer charities called immediately for better research rather than simply demanding immediate prescriptions. One was the small Challenge Breast Cancer in Scotland, the other was a charity in New Zealand, the Auckland Women's Health Council, which said:

'The Council continues to advocate for an evidence based approach to be taken regarding the use of Herceptin while the results from the drug trials are gathered and fully reported upon. The controversy over access to this drug and the best treatment regime being argued for by both the drug's manufacturer and breast cancer groups continues to obscure the facts and has lead [sic] to a narrow focus on the cost of the drug for patients and the concurrent demand for public funding.'[11]

Neither take any pharmaceutical funding.

Patients' groups and lucre

Money. Where it comes from is important. As we have seen, even small gifts from drug companies to doctors can change the way they prescribe, even if the doctors don't think so. We are not good at telling when we are influenced. We can easily lack insight into our own behaviour.

This is dangerous territory. Insight keeps us independent, critical, and safe from vested interests.

Can we even tell which healthcare charities are taking money from pharmaceutical companies? Sometimes we can. The British Skin Foundation is supported by several pharmaceutical companies, including Dermal Laboratories Ltd and Typharm,[12] as well as commercial skincare products such as Veet, and Dr Nick Lowe, who markets various skincare products, such as 'Dark Circles Correcting Cream' and 'Lifting Super Serum'.[13] Heart UK, which styles itself 'The Cholesterol Charity', has accepted funds from AstraZeneca, Boehringer-Ingelheim and Sanofi-Aventis, among others, as well as the manufacturers of Flora pro.activ margarine and Kellogg's Optivita, a cereal 'specifically developed with oat bran to help lower cholesterol'.[14] The IBS Network, which is the 'charity for people with irritable bowel syndrome', has as 'partners' Norgine, a pharmaceutical company, as well as Danone and Yakult, yogurt makers.[15] Breakthrough Breast Cancer encourages what it calls a 'marketing partnership' with organisations such as Marks and Spencer and hair straighteners company ghd, saying that this can deliver:

'. . . increased sales, access to new markets, positive PR coverage, emotionalise a brand, create an experience, delivering on CSR [corporate social responsibility] goals. How could this work? Create a new pink product, or turn an existing product pink, with a donation to Breakthrough. Educate staff and customers about the importance of being breast aware. Hold a pink fund raising day, or week, or even month, to raise vital funds.'[16]

Accounts from Breakthrough disclose funding from pharmaceutical companies Pfizer, Roche and Novartis.[17] The funding included sending staff to a medical conference in the US. It is only when you look up the annual report of Parkinson's UK that funds from Boehringer-Ingelheim, Genus Pharmaceuticals, GlaxoSmithKline, Orion and Norgine are listed.[18] Asthma UK works with GlaxoSmithKline, which has provided funding for asthma nurses, conferences and honoraria to the chief executive of Asthma UK.[19] They say they have created a 'level playing field' by allowing AstraZeneca UK, GlaxoSmithKline and NAPP 'corporate gold' membership.[20]

An interesting relationship exists at Diabetes UK, which runs an annual conference for healthcare professionals and suggests they fund their attendance via pharma. 'Funding for educational conferences can be obtained via your pharmaceutical representative . . . once you have received confirmation that your pharmaceutical representative will be able to fund all or part of your registration fee, we can either send an invoice to your rep, pay via their credit card online or send a cheque in the post.'[21] GSK lists during 2010, £40,000 to sponsor a Young Diabetologists Forum meeting, registration fees for the Diabetes UK conference, and, during 2009, £4,000 for 'speakers' honoraria, venue and catering costs' for a conference.[22] Just in case you were wondering, 'honoraria' is another way of saying 'fees'.

There is no better way to illustrate the workings of charities, PR and pharma than with an apparently spontaneous uprising over generic drugs. The Department of Health had proposed that pharmacists should be allowed to change prescriptions for branded (more expensive) medicines to generic, and therefore cheaper, ones. Generally, drugs come off patent at about seven years, which means that a previously branded medication can be manufactured without the manufacturer's trade name and by another company. This usually means plainer packaging and savings to the NHS. During the consultation process, a letter appeared in the *Times* newspaper in 2010 entitled 'Patient wellbeing at risk from substituted generic medicines'.[23] It was signed by a number of patient groups including the British Liver Trust, the Cure Parkinsons' Trust, and The British Cardiac Patients Association. They called for the Department of Health, to 'respect the judgment of the prescriber'. However, it transpired that the letter, which would have been read by many people being prescribed generic or branded medication for illnesses, was instigated by a PR company, Burson-Marsteller. This company evidently trawled the medical press for signs of doctors with doubts about prescribing generics, and funded a meeting of these doctors, together with representatives of the charities they had contacted and some journalists – expenses paid – and then co-ordinated the signing of the letter by all. Who paid for the PR company? Norgine, a pharmaceutical company. Norgine's chief operating officer did not sign his name, and he explained why to me: 'Having a pharmaceutical company in there would sully the message.'[24]

Are patient groups and charities in as much danger of bias as doctors when they liaise with pharmaceutical companies? A group of researchers examined 69 patient organisations for details of possible funding from pharma. Only a third were clear on where their money came from and just four said they had an advertising and conflict of interest policy.[25] In Amsterdam, researchers found that only one in 20 patient organisations was opposed to pharmaceutical sponsorship.[26] In the UK, researchers have found that, of 126 organisations who replied to their questions, just 26% who were known to be receiving pharmaceutical funding or support openly acknowledged it.[27]

At the very least, we should be able to judge for ourselves whose information we want to trust. We can't do that if we don't know what influences might have exerted themselves over that information. And what about the delivery of that information itself? Do we really want to be confronted with the 'emotionalisation' of cancer when we buy a bra or a T-shirt, or for a brand's need for 'CSR' to dictate what we are told about cancer, cholesterol or Parkinson's disease?

The uprising of 'awareness'

Healthcare charities have positioned themselves as the advocates of patients and their families. They have taken a lead role not just in political campaigning but also in 'awareness'.

What harm could this do? How, possibly, could one argue that ignorance is better than 'awareness'? Unfortunately, the motivation and practice of raising awareness leads directly to overinflated claims and hype. The sexing up of medicine has roots in this culture of awareness.

One of the very biggest problems has been the assumption that awareness is good. This is made, almost uniformly, by health charities wanting to promote their cause. Only rarely – and even then, it is usually tangentially – is there any examination of the potential harms of such an unswerving drive.

As a GP, I know these harms exist. I see them, from the sleepless teenager terrified that her (normal) developing breast is actually cancer, to the man who is embarrassed that he has 'waited so long' to get his testicular lump seen to. It is difficult to appreciate the problems – anxiety, misinformation, distress – that 'awareness' can inadvertently bring. You need hard-nosed, unemotional assessments of what good, and bad, awareness campaigns can cause. Ostensibly well-meaning campaigns have gone woefully under-examined for their side-effects. It is an enormous, collective blind spot.

Nothing seems too much when it comes to awareness. The 'CoppaFeel!' charity aims to 'hit home the importance of breast examination in younger women' with its mission to 'make Brits boob aware by "hijacking" everyone and everything in sight with CoppaFeel! stickers; and get them copping-a-feel!' Giant breasts were used to attract attention from passers-by. If women notice anything abnormal, they are advised to see their GP and 'demand action.'[28] The Male Cancer Awareness Campaign says: 'We don't do research as we believe that education is the key in the fight against male cancer . . . we raise awareness all the year round.' Its aims include: 'To increase awareness of how to detect the symptoms of cancer in the early stages' and for 'education on the early warning signs of male cancer' to become 'part of the national school curriculum.'[29] To do this, the charity uses a character called Mr Testicles and 'near naked men' who have been photographed in the name of awareness together with at least one MP at the Houses of Parliament.[30] Orchid, a charity whose strapline is 'fighting male cancer' says 'Know your balls . . . check 'em out', advising that 'many men are unaware of testicular cancer, or prefer to ignore it, and that few people check their testicles.'[31]

Macmillan Cancer Support tells men that from 'puberty onwards, it's important that men check their testicles regularly (once a month) for anything unusual like a lump or a swelling.'[32] Television programmes have featured doctors demonstrating the 'correct' way to self-examine the scrotal sac. This, along with the avalanche of 'cancer awareness' stickers, T-shirts, bubble baths, leaflets, websites and media coverage, means average citizens do well to escape having their awareness raised, whether they like it or not.

Does awareness work?

Medicine, as we have seen, does not always work to what might be considered sensible and logical deductions. You can have pet theories about which way to lay children down to sleep or which drugs to give people with head injuries. But unless you have good evidence – unless you can say that you have decent proof – you have no idea if you are doing more harm than good.

This is not a nice thing to contemplate. Many people who have been motivated to set up a health charity and to campaign for 'more' have been people who, in one way or another, have been affected by the issues they want to make a noise about. Some of that is absolutely understandable and some might even be useful. But we cannot assume that all will be good. We need evidence. When charities say 'check your balls once a month' or 'touch, feel, check!' we need to be sure that this is a good idea – even though it sounds like it is.

Errors in awareness

After 30 years of pink crusading, one might expect that at the very least we might be a bit more knowledgeable about breast cancer. Alas, this is not the case. It could be argued that despite – or even *because of* – the publicity attached to it, we are less well educated and more frightened about it.

Let's take the headline figure of 'One in eight women will get breast cancer' which is a number generated by Cancer Research UK, and agreed with breast cancer charities. This number is quoted on websites and in publicity material. These 'lifetime risks' of getting breast cancer have been advertised on buses, taxis, and advertising hoardings over the past decade by a mixture of charities and healthcare organisations. It is a short, succinct, and bite-sized statistic, readily understood. But it is also misleading and inaccurate. 'One in eight' is a measurement of lifetime risk. The 'lifetime' assumes women live to the age of 85, but since most women in the UK die before this, the risk automatically becomes an overestimation.

We also know that as a result of breast screening, more women are being diagnosed with a breast cancer that would never have maimed or killed them (see Part One.) So we are finding more breast cancers just because we are using screening mammography to pick them up but we are not necessarily finding them *usefully*. We are diagnosing more cancers but these are not always cancers that are going to maim or kill.

The most recent calculations on breast cancer risk in the UK publicised the fact that breast cancer risk had increased from one in nine to one in eight. This has the appearance of a large shift, from an 11.1% chance to a new higher 12.5% chance. Yet because the numbers on risk have been rounded up by Cancer Research UK, the shift in risk over the past few years has been much smaller and slower. In 2004, the lifetime chance of getting breast cancer was 12.09%. The same comparative figure for 2008 – the last data available – was 12.51%. So sure, yes, a rise: but a rise of 0.42% over that period.[33]

'Lifetime risk' is a sexed-up number that does not give us a good handle on what our risks are. Indeed, an article in the *New England Journal of Medicine* criticised the handling of data using lifetime risk scores:

> 'Although breast cancer is an important cause of premature death, its incidence is approximately equivalent to that of lung cancer (a predominantly preventable disease) and vastly smaller than that of cardiovascular disease. . . These facts are not well understood by the public . . . The media have had a central role in communicating information about the risk of breast cancer, particularly in disseminating the one in nine statistic. The focus on this statistic, especially when it is sometimes linked to images of young women with incurable stages of the disease, can distort the public's perception of the risk.'[34]

And indeed, women do overestimate their risk of getting breast cancer. Despite most women knowing about breast cancer, 80% of women overestimated their risk of getting breast cancer[35] and only 1% of women have been found to correctly estimate their risk in relation to age.[36] This sounds to me like women are being alarmed, not informed.

What about Mr Testicles? Has he been enough to educate men fairly? There is a large gap in evidence. We do not know if men are being usefully informed about testicular cancer and risks; we do know that there are dozens of men's health charities promoting testicular awareness but far fewer visible campaigns on the larger risks to men's health such as smoking, alcohol excess or road traffic accidents. Some studies suggest that men are unaware of the 'importance' of testicular self-examination[37,38] and offer this as evidence to campaign more on the subject. However, it is clear that despite this, testicular cancer remains, overall, rare and most men with testicular cancer do not die from it. In 2008, the last available figures, 2,138 men were diagnosed with testicular cancer in the UK; just 70 died from it.[39]

If testicular awareness were being funded by the taxpayer, we would have a right to expect that the outcomes of it were fairly investigated by good research and that we would know whether or not to recommend it. We would be advancing knowledge, ensuring that we did not waste time and effort – and that we did not do harm. Research is, quite rightly, audited and reviewed; the firmness of evidence is up for discussion and debate.

Some healthcare charities do get governmental grants. Many rely on donations from the public. But if you are being alarmed or scared into believing that a disease is more common than it really is, and if you are prepared to fund a charity on that basis, there is little motivation for a charity to examine its own prejudices, or even the evidence for its powerful authority.

The spiral, the quadratic, and the mystic

Aberdeen, circa 1993: divide the breast into quadrants in order to examine it properly. As a final year medical student, I was told to examine each mammary gland like this, using a two-handed approach. I was told to tell women to do this regularly themselves.

Aberdeen, circa 2001: now we should examine the breast in a spiral, starting from the nipple and working our way around. This wasn't just for women who came to their doctor having noticed, by themselves, a breast lump. No, this was women who were perfectly well, but whose doctor thought it was a good idea to check their breasts because, say, they were on the Pill, which increases breast cancer risk. And anyway, it was a good opportunity to teach women how to do breast self-examination. Doctors, since the patient was naked from the waist up, could use this moment to ensure that the patient got it right when it came to monthly self-examination. I took this opportunity for preventive medicine seriously. I examined, instructed and motivated dutifully.

There was a nagging feeling of unease. Was I really doing this the right way? I took it upon myself to find every leaflet I could, from Cancer Research UK, to Breakthrough Breast Cancer, instructing women on how to self-examine their breasts. I found pink diagrams of women with hands on hips, hands behind heads, lying down, standing up, poking, prodding, rolling and patting themselves. Which was the right way to do it?

The penny slowly dropped. There was no 'right way'. The reason that there were so many opinions on how to examine breasts was that no one had tested them. We were wading about in an ignorant gloop consisting of whim and opinion, not evidence. No surprise that women were getting conflicting instructions. Doctors were being told to encourage self-examination without a clear idea of what this actually consisted of or even whether teaching women to do this was a good thing.

Medicine likes to think of itself as a useful and powerful force for good. But you have to know that you really are 'good'. It is easier to do things than not to – harder to sit on hands than it is to write a prescription. The authority of medicine enjoys displays of instruction and activity; it is so much harder to question and doubt it.

When the US National Cancer Institute instigated a trial in China to see if teaching women breast self-examination was useful in preventing deaths from breast cancer, it was courageously questioning a 'truth' that had been propagated worldwide by doctors, breast cancer care charities and nurses who had all thought they were doing the right thing.

The study took more than a quarter of a million Chinese women and divided them into two groups. One group was taught how to examine their breasts and then reminded to do so monthly, as well as being medically supervised for their examinations every six months. The other group acted as a control group, and they were not taught, or reminded, to examine their breasts. At the end of the study, there had been similar amounts of breast cancer diagnosed in each group and similar numbers of deaths from breast cancer. The theory was wrong: teaching and encouraging women to do breast self-examination did not stop women dying from breast cancer. In fact, women doing breast self-exams ended up having more biopsies for benign, non-cancerous lumps. It could even be considered that self-examination did more harm than good. The study, published in 2002, concluded: 'Women who choose to practice breast self-examination should be informed that its efficacy is unproven and that it may increase their chances of having a benign breast biopsy.'[40]

What about testicular examination? Multiple, determined campaigns insist that men should examine their testicles monthly. Online video tutorials on the order of feeling and squeezing scrotums insist that the right way is theirs and that this is an essential regular health check for all men.

Deaths from testicular cancer are relatively rare. The 70 deaths in the UK in 2008 represented a death rate of 0.2 per 100,000.[41] Deaths from testicular cancer have been falling nicely since the 1970s. Compare this to the suicide rate of men aged between 15 and 44, which is just under 18 per 100,000 population – almost a hundred times more. Suicide is a much more common cause of male death than testicular cancer.[42] Globally, road traffic crashes are the leading cause of death in young people.[43]

Our perceptions of what might harm or maim us become skewed instead by what is popular; there are few campaigns by charity groups keen to increase 'awareness' of suicide or the disproportionate burden of young male deaths in car accidents.

This is one of the great problems with awareness – what we become aware of depends on how popular a cause can become. Pop star Rachel Stevens appeared in a 'cheeky new Everyman advertisement aimed at making men sit up and take notice of the warning signs of testicular cancer. . . Rachel's alluring invitation asks men to put their hands down their trousers as she explains exactly what they should be looking for and the best way to check themselves.' Rachel, posing lasciviously on a bed, toys with a couple of plums and tells the press 'it's a fun way of raising awareness.'[44] Would mental health advice be given the same treatment? I doubt it.

It just doesn't add up to healthy perceptions of risk. With The Male Cancer Awareness Charity telling us that we don't need research, just awareness, it's not surprising that the belief that checking your body regularly is good for you has become ingrained as a certainty when it is nothing of the sort. The subtle truth is being disregarded. Men are usually aware when they have a testicular lump. Just like women and their breasts, or legs or arms or skin or nose or knees, we wash, bathe, shower, dress and notice our bodies. Men notice when something is wrong. The issue is that when men notice something is wrong, they often take rather a long time to get advice about it. This may have improved over the past decade; in 1987 it was common for men who knew they had a testicular lump to wait for six months before seeing a doctor.[45] One UK study found that, in Yorkshire, the time taken for men to seek advice about a lump has decreased over time, from 14 weeks in 1985 to two weeks in 2002.[46]

Yet this improvement in the time taken for men to get medical advice has happened without the uptake of advice to perform regular testicular self-examination. The vast majority of men don't practise self-examination, but most have heard about testicular cancer.[47] This squares with my experience as a doctor: I have yet to have a man come in to tell me about his testicular symptoms who isn't terrified of cancer. While cancer charities are keen to encourage testicular self-examination, they are less keen to publicise the fact that testicular cancer, one of the highly treatable forms of cancer and considered to be curable, need not be a major cause of terror. Rather than accusing men of being 'totally ignorant' about the disease,[48] it would be evidence based and more informative if men were reminded that any lump should be seen promptly by a doctor. Men are not told, amid the rough and tumble creation of catchphrases and publicity stunts, that deaths from testicular cancer are rare, testicular cancer is treatable and that a cancerous lump is far less common than a benign one. A very small but detailed study in the journal *Psycho-oncology* found one rare patient who did practise regular self-examination and found a lump. He still did not seek advice for six months: fear of cancer and surgery contributed to the timing of other men seeking advice.[49] We cannot assume that 'awareness' will lead to useful changes in our behaviour.

This is the worst thing about the cult of awareness. It does not mean education, designed to impart knowledge and understanding. It is awareness designed to attract attention, alarm and publicity, which often ripples panic and bad statistics in its wake.

In light of the China breast self-examination study, which showed that teaching women to do self-examination was, if anything, harmful, most breast cancer charities tried to acknowledge this finding. Did they do enough? Instead of setting up trials to test what advice would be best for women, most breast cancer charities advocate 'TLC: Touch, look, check'. This seems rather a fudge. Breakthrough Breast Cancer says that there is no single recommended way to self-examine breasts, and offers advice to 'be thorough when checking your breasts . . . check your breasts regularly so you get to know how they look and feel at different times of the month'.[50] Rather than trying to get better information about what advice would be best for women, we have become stuck on the idea that awareness and self-examination are for the best.

Know your prostate

The Prostate Cancer Charity has decreed that its Awareness Month shall now cover the whole of March. They state: 'All men are entitled to have the test on the NHS if they want it.'[51] After the National Screening Committee looked at the evidence for PSA testing in 2010, and decided that a screening programme would not be useful, the chief executive of the charity wrote in a newspaper that:

'It's far too controversial to be nailed on the basis of the committee's narrowly focused review . . . the critical flip-side, which is heavily underplayed in the screening committee's announcement, is that for some men with an aggressive and symptomless prostate cancer, a raised PSA level may be the only earlier indicator of a cancer at a time when it can be successfully treated. PSA testing is a two way street. It has pros. It has cons. But until an improved test is developed, it is the best we have . . . Here, we come to the scandalous reality. The government, through its Prostate Cancer Risk Management Programme says that every man over 50 who doesn't have symptoms of prostate cancer is entitled to ask his GP for a PSA test. Yet, 70% of men don't even know that the test exists, let alone their right to request it – men are effectively denied the right to make a choice.'[52]

The Prostate Screening Trust states:

'Don't sit on the problem, have a PSA blood test. Ask your doctor for a simple blood test it only takes ten minutes . . . Our aim will be to show that regular blood testing will pick up possible cancer activity through PSA levels.'[53]

Is this fair to men wanting high-quality information about prostate cancer screening? The steer is of entitlement; men being denied a potentially life-saving intervention is presented as the worst possible scenario. But is it? What about the scenario of having had invasive surgery for a prostate cancer that was never going to kill you, or having surgery with complications of impotence or incontinence, which have been noted in 88% and 66% respectively of men after such surgery?[54]

The Prostate Cancer Federation, a group of charities interested in the disease, decided that when, as expected, the National Screening Committee did not recommend PSA screening, it would 'lobby government to implement alternative arrangements for "universal informed choice" e.g. through routine "well man" health checks'.[34]

But what happens when you get better, fairer information? Scientists who deal with the explanation of risk have noticed a trend. When you supply better information to people about prostate screening, you do not increase uptake of the test. Better information means that fewer men want it done.

A systematic review examined the effect on men's choices of 'decision aids' – formal written or online information about the pros and cons of the PSA test, to use either alone or with a healthcare professional. It was found, and this was consistent with previous reviews in this area, that such decision aids made men more knowledgeable and more confident about the decisions they made. However, men also chose less PSA screening, and more 'watchful waiting' – avoiding surgery or invasive treatment – rather than operative treatment if they did go on to have a PSA screening test.[55] A US study – where PSA screening is part of standard Medicare testing – examined the relationship between prostate screening and information. At the start, almost all men – 97% – wanted PSA screening. But when men were given a video and a discussion about the pros and cons, only half the men wanted to proceed with it.[56]

Alas, we don't know what would happen if the equivalent decent information was shared with women being sent appointments for cervical or breast screening; the same kind of research hasn't been done. But the fact remains that giving people better information about medical tests may result in fewer rather than more tests being done.

If a charity has founded itself on the principle that more screening is better, it may be rather difficult for that charity to question either the test, or information that might make people want the test less.

The function of many charities is not to ensure that people get high-quality information about medical interventions. Instead, their rallying cry is for attention. There was no mention of false positives, unnecessary treatments, or debate over PSA testing in a leaflet the Prostate Cancer Campaign sent out (with the support of the drug company AstraZeneca), which was not aimed at men, but at women. It recommended, with the aim of getting him to the doctor 'to discuss prostate health' that the woman of the house should 'tug at his heartstrings: "do it for me/us/the family, as it means such a lot" or "use friends' experience as examples of times when a trip to the doctor resulted in peace of mind or a successful outcome".[57] This information is biased and incomplete. We deserve better.

Awareness, with its emphasis on slick slogans and PR messages instead of research and evidence-based actions, is truly an example of sexed-up medicine in action.

11

The problem with PR

In 2006, an advert appeared in the back pages of the *Guardian* newspaper.

> 'Finger on the pulse?' it read. 'Celebrity booker – attractive salary plus benefits . . . Do you know who's hot and who's not in the world of celebrity? . . . Working in partnership with our current celebrity supporter manager, the successful candidate will help us secure an impressive array of high-profile individuals to support the charity. . . You will be well connected, able to influence, persuade, cajole and 'schmooze' the busiest of agents and celebrities. You will be seen at all the right events and all the right places, and your connection, passion and drive will deliver results.'[1]

Indeed, in another recent advert, the same charity – the British Heart Foundation – was not looking for someone with scientific credentials to man the out-of-hours press contact phone number, but someone with a 'solid knowledge of celebrity media and a strong list of contacts'.[2]

Celebrities who get involved with charities may have profoundly good motives for doing so. But it is also obvious that some famous people have ulterior motives – publicity for their own books or films. Some celebrities might just have been charmed into it by a 'celebrity booker'.

The problem is that if charities want to give us good information about our health then we have to be able to trust them to do so. If we as consumers find that our information is being served to us courtesy of schmoozing rather than facts, we have a right to question its reliability.

The same charity launched its 'Mending broken hearts' campaign in 2011, designed to raise £50 million towards researching the cardiovascular system of the zebrafish. The BHF said its research 'could begin to "mend broken hearts" in as little as ten years' time . . . our exciting news has made headlines in lots of today's national papers, radio and TV bulletins and across the internet'. Celebrities added their weight to the BHF's obvious pride in the media attention it had generated.[3] Reports of a 'pill that allows damaged hearts to repair themselves could be available in as little as seven years'[4] were based on BHF's own literature, with reports saying 'British scientists create miracle pill to mend broken hearts.'[5] Indeed, the BHF's medical director was quoted as saying: 'We really could make recovering from a heart attack as simple as getting over a broken leg.'[6]

Yet underneath the BHF's headline of 'It's not science fiction' came the inevitable rider: 'Within five years we hope to begin early clinical trials. Within ten years we aim to be running full trials. Within a further decade, people living with heart failure could look forward to a brighter future.'[7]

A little bit of arithmetic reveals a truth rather contrary to that singing from the headlines: 20 years might – might – see the availability of a medication resulting from the research programme. Not five years, not seven: 20.

Alas, it seems that the mission the BHF gave the media was not to disseminate fair information about the work it wished the public to fund but instead to create a hype: a disproportionately optimistic version of the slow, tedious reality of medical research.

People wishing to support the research are given high expectations of when and what will be achieved, while the opportunity to be involved with a realistic appraisal of how scientific research is done is missed entirely. Miraculous but currently fictional cures are created out of newspaper inches; with such an unclear presentation of how research is done, patient expectations are inflated beyond reality.

Darth Vader does prostates

Earlier chapters described the impact of charities such as Jo's Trust on the submissions to the government on cervical cancer screening, which were not based in evidence. The awareness campaigns from many breast cancer charities are likely to have contributed to the misunderstandings many people have about it.

Charities are competitive. Success is not measured in accuracy, the acknowledgement of uncertainty or the provision of unbiased information. It's measured in column inches. So if you can, get the actor who played Darth Vader, and who supports the Prostate Cancer Charity, to say to his fans at Star Wars conventions: 'I ask the gentlemen in the audience if they have been tested for prostate cancer . . . If they don't put their hands up, I tell them, very politely, to go and get checked . . . I explain that I was tested almost on a whim. And that whim saved my life.'[8] No mention, naturally, of the evidence base, of false positives or the potential harms of unnecessary surgery.

If doctors give out health information and it is wrong, they are rightly challenged by their peers and, if necessary, their regulator in the UK, the General Medical Council. Celebrities have no such checks. So when 'spokesmodel' Elizabeth Hurley, representing the Estée Lauder Breast Cancer Campaign, says that 'We should tell every woman we know — whether our mother, grandmother, sister, daughter or girlfriend — that it is very important to check their breasts and that they need to go to their doctors for a mammogram every year, if they are over the age of 40. Don't leave it for an extra year, because if you get a mammogram once a year, at the very latest your cancer is only 364 days old,'[9] or Net-a-Porter's Natalie Massenet tells her audience that 'one in four women get breast cancer',[10] we enter an unregulated realm.

Advertising health doesn't produce fair results, even with good intentions. Instead, advertising, twinned with public relations, stage manages and distorts decent health information.

When charities approve of products

Product placement in the cinema or soap operas is generally greeted with cynicism on behalf of viewers who don't like the idea that they are being manipulated. What happens, though, when it is not a hotel chain or a computer manufacturer being given approval, but a product being sold for your health?

Heart UK is 'passionate about preventing premature deaths caused by high cholesterol and cardiovascular disease'. Heart UK's partners include Flora pro-activ, Kellogg's Optivita, Nestlé Shredded Wheat, Welch's Purple Grape Juice, and Hovis Hearty Oats. In its accounts, Heart UK lists 'product approval licence fees' as a significant annual income.[11] It offers to allow commercial companies to add its logo to their products in order to:

> 'Identify and draw attention to foods and food products that may have beneficial effects on the causes of and contributors to cardiovascular disease, including raised cholesterol, thus providing helpful information to the public . . . Consumers can be assured that the nature of the product and evidence supporting the claim have been reviewed by members of Heart UK's Product Approval Working Group. . . Heart UK levies a non-returnable product approval application fee of £1,000 to cover the initial evaluation work involved. There may be additional costs, depending on the complexity of the evaluation according to product type.'[12]

And customers also might like to know that 'Heart UK works in partnership with a broad representation of organisations to help achieve its campaigning objectives.' The charity, as we've already noted, is partnered with companies making goods from margarine to statins.

I'm not at all sure this is such a 'service'. Why should we think that branded shredded wheat is better than a cheaper own brand? Where are the approval stickers on plain apples and bananas, which evidence shows are good for our health but which don't have any brand or marketers of their own to request approval? Aren't customers going to be pointed towards only those brands that are rich enough and PR astute enough to concentrate on image? If we are going to be 'helped' to healthier lives through the efforts of PR companies, we are likely to get a raw deal.

PR and scientists

One of the joys of being on press lists is getting missives from the PR industry. Public relations professionals are not just the keepers of celebrity and the famous. PR departments are also an integral part of universities and NHS research units, as well as pharmaceutical companies and many healthcare charities. Perhaps there were good intentions to begin with: perhaps, as the PR industry was birthed and grew, it was hoped that helping journalists to obtain good facts and discuss published, or about-to-be-published, results with scientists, could improve health reporting or provide useful insights.

There are some nice people working in PR and press offices around the country but they don't often help me to make newspaper articles better. Instead, press offices want to control who you can speak to, coach those people in what they should say, and will only publicise certain papers while disregarding others. Press notices consist of information their writers desire that you know, rather than what you perhaps *should* know.

Let's take the press release from the WOSCOPS study (West of Scotland Coronary Prevention Study), mentioned earlier, which resulted in worldwide media coverage in 1995. The headline was:

'Landmark study: Pravastatin rapidly reduces risk of heart attacks and saves lives of people with high cholesterol and no previous heart attack.'

This was one of the very first statin primary prevention studies, which would eventually lead to the current practice of risk managing most middle-aged adults for vascular risk. Were the headlines correct? Yes. But they were also guilty of overselling their results. The press release continues:

'People with high cholesterol can rapidly reduce their risk of having a first-time heart attack by 31% and their risk of death by 22%, by taking a widely prescribed drug called pravastatin sodium. This is the conclusion of a landmark study presented today at the annual meeting of the American Heart Association. The results . . . found that treatment with pravastatin reduced the risk of first-time heart attack and death . . . WOSCOPS extends the evidence to show that pravastatin provides early, sustained and significant reductions in cardiovascular disease and death in patients with elevated cholesterol but without previous heart attack.'

The press release finished off with a table of numbers and a quote.

Event	Risk reduction	Statistical significance
Nonfatal heart attack or death from heart disease	31%	p = 0.0001
Heart attack	31%	p = 0.0005
Revascularisation procedures	37%	p = 0.009
Death from cardiovascular causes	32%	p = 0.033
Death from any cause	22%	p = 0.051*

* When adjusted for baseline risk factors, risk reduction equals 24% (p = 0.039)

'These are some of the most striking data I have ever seen in heart attack and total mortality reduction,' said Professor Shepherd. 'The findings strongly support current treatment guidelines and irrefutably encourage physicians to actively treat people who are at risk for a heart attack,' he added.[13]

Doesn't it look impressive? A reduction in risk of heart attacks of 31% and a reduction in death of 32%. No wonder Professor Shepherd (the principal trial investigator) says it's 'the most striking data' he's ever seen. Except that all these numbers are relative risks, not absolute risks. As we've seen, these can be misleading. If you can cut a risk of a disease from two in a million to one in a million, you are entitled to say that you have cut the risk in half – this is the relative risk. If, though, you give the absolute risk, you will simply say that you can reduce the risk of a disease from two in a million to one in a million. In this way you are explaining more about how likely people are to benefit from your treatment. The absolute risk looks like a less impressive number but it is also a more helpful number. You can see right away how the treatment looks in context and what the chances of avoiding a heart attack or death with pravastatin are.

The absolute risk reduction with pravastatin is not so impressive. The trial ran over five years. In the WOSCOPS placebo group of 3,293 men, 135 died from any cause. In the pravastatin group of 3,302 men, there were 106 deaths. This means that 4.09% of men died in the placebo group compared with 3.21% in the pravastatin group. Therefore, if you take pravastatin, the reduction in your risk of death, expressed as absolute risk, falls from 4.09% to 3.21%.[14]

Sure, it's a reduction in risk. You can see how you could use the same facts to push a person into taking the tablets or not. After WOSCOPs was published in the *New England Journal of Medicine*, adverts started to appear encouraging doctors to prescribe pravastatin in patients who had been considered at low risk of heart attacks and strokes. A psychologist wrote in the *BMJ* about another way of expressing the known facts about pravastatin:

'Medicine is not an exact science. Therefore, 200 men without any prior heart disease have to swallow 357,700 tablets over five years to save one of them dying from coronary heart disease. This is due to the fact that no exact knowledge exists as to whom of these 200 will benefit from treatment.'[15]

How do I, as a doctor, make sure that I am giving my patients unbiased advice about whether to take a statin or not? Some doctors would say that we are not using enough in the way of statins or other preventive medicine in low-risk patients. For example, one group of researchers invented, in 2003, a 'polypill' – with the intention that it be used for large sections of the population, no matter how high or low their individual risk.[16] Richard Smith, then editor of the *BMJ*, published the paper-based (not patient-based) and theoretical proposal with the headline: 'The most important *BMJ* for 50 years?'[17]

The small overall benefits that patients may get from preventive medication are pushed into the limelight where wondrous things are meant to happen. This may be okay, even very good, if you were in the WOSCOPS trial and among that 0.88% of people taking a statin whose death was delayed because of it. But what about the people who had intolerable side-effects and stopped taking it and who have worried about their inability to take the tablets every day since?

The other problem that occurs when preventive measures are applied to people in their millions is that the numbers of uncommon and rare side-effects start to stack up. We've already discussed the issue with diabetes risk. A large study, which collected data about patients prescribed statins, reported, in 2010 that there were small increased risks of liver dysfunction, kidney failure, moderate or serious myopathy (muscle inflammation) and cataract.[18] If patients are going to get good information about drugs they need to know about adverse effects too.

Press releases like the one heralding the WOSCOPS trial remind me more of adverts than of fair information. Does this approach serve the needs of doctors and patients? Sadly, most days there is something in my inbox that makes me worry that medical journals present their findings so as to attract any sort of attention.

So, 'Flash!' reads a press release, fluttering into prime email inbox position: 'Could sage be the new superfood?'

Tempting as it is to dismiss the non-scientific moniker 'superfood' as the nonsense PR it is (we need mixed, balanced diets; there is no substitute for variety) let us concentrate on where this press release came from. The owners of vast sage plantations? Supermarkets planning to devote a whole aisle to sage-based products? No. It came from the publishing house of Elsevier, purveyors of the highly esteemed medical journal, the *Lancet*.

Information followed: a new study published in Elsevier's *Fitoterapia* evaluates the anti-ulcerogenic activity of the hydroalcoholic (HO) extract of (sage)'. But the study was not in humans, but rats. Sage seemed to reduce the size of some of the ulcers that had been artificially created.

So Elsevier sent out a press release asking whether sage was the new superfood, based on research showing that you could give rats slightly less large stomach ulcers if you also gave them sage. Not only was this a small, animal- and laboratory-based study with no human subjects in sight, it had not even used sage in dietary form.[19]

The fault is not the study, which is scientifically fair enough, but the silly extrapolation. Who wrote the headline? 'Our PR agency researches and writes the synopses,' said the press team. 'The Elsevier press office then approves the synopses and also requests approval from publishing editors and authors before it is included in one of the ['newsflash!'] editions.'

So the publishing company's press office franchises out the writing of synopses to a PR agency with the intention of making the stories as sellable as possible. (Elsevier said the phrase 'Is sage the new superfood?' was thrown in separately, however, to 'add editorial interest').[20] So the scientists who actually did the study are relegated to third-hand tellers of their story. The researchers should, of course, insist on a fact-based press release. When a PR company working for the journal is asked to generate heat first, not light, a conflict of interest appears for researchers who are pushed towards a sexed-up, and potentially misleading, version of their work.

So, healthcare charities, medical journals, and PR departments offer information that may or may not be influenced by a need for publicity, or the pharmaceutical industry, and that may or may not be based on fair evidence.

It's tempting, then, to hope that getting to the source – the actual science itself – will reliably reveal sense.

Indeed. Go to the websites of many academic journals and you will find paywalls rising up at most of your clicks to get to the paper behind them. Most medical journals require subscription. There is an inherent ethical problem here: when people take part in research studies, they should be able to expect that the results of those studies are made widely available. For example, if a study is done showing that a drug has serious side-effects and no benefits, it would be important that this result was widely available to prevent further trials of this drug being done. Paywalls mean this isn't guaranteed to happen. It's true, though, that many medical editors are aware of this problem and various enterprises to enable free access to journals – or some content of journals – have begun. One model is that publication is costed in the original proposal, and dissemination of findings becomes part of the research stipulation. While this is desirable, it is relatively rare, and the majority of research is for those with either personal or academic subscriptions. Papers generally cost $40 or $50 each to view. Abstracts – a summary of the paper – are usually available for free. However, abstracts are not reliable sources of information about the study. For example, one team examined scientific papers where the result was not 'statistically significant' – their result was not reliable enough to exclude chance as the cause of the result. The team concluded that 'the reporting and interpretation of findings was frequently inconsistent with the results.'[21] Another paper found that trial abstracts reported the statistical workings of the research a minority of the time, with only half the abstracts reporting side-effects or harms from the intervention.[22]

'The media' are often decried as poor ambassadors of science and, certainly, there are a lot of bad headlines in the press and poor relaying of research findings to readers. The UK parliamentary Select Committee on Science and Technology found, in 2000, that 'many scientists are convinced that science is treated badly by the media.'[23]

But whose fault is this? One can't ignore the slew of over-excited press releases coming from academic journals and the science departments of universities and research institutions. What if it is not the press who are inflating tentative research findings but researchers themselves who are overselling their work?

The *Annals of Internal Medicine* reported a series of 200 press releases from medical centres in both high- and low-rated institutions: 74% of animal studies claimed a relevance to human health; 23% didn't mention study size and 34% didn't quantify their results.[24] The report concluded that: 'Academic center press releases often promote research with uncertain clinical relevance without emphasising important cautions or limitations.'

We have also seen how the use of relative risks rather than absolute risks can distort our perception of how useful a treatment is. Press reports about a new treatment or intervention do not routinely include information about who might have a vested interest in the research being promoted.[25] Unfortunately, the misdemeanours of the press release, for which academics have to take responsibility, have largely gone unnoticed in the UK.

Blaming the press for bad science stories does not get to the heart of the problem. Instead, it is scientists who may present, or be colluding to present, their stories in a way that emphasises the speculative. Is science by press release really a fair way to inform people about new discoveries and potential therapies?

For all its faults, the NHS at least attempts to assess what treatments and interventions there is evidence for, and to provide healthcare based on that evidence. The process of healthcare within the NHS is audited; doctors' prescribing habits are open to scrutiny. When you leave the NHS behind, the healthcare marketplace turns treacherous – a minefield of competing claims. PR companies and advertising rule the information. For prospective patients, this is bad news.

Pure PR

Fancy a night out? How about one that provides women 'with fashion and style advice', an 'inspirational class providing top tips on how to rejuvenate your beauty routine' and the opportunity to rediscover that 'spark in their love lives'. The developers of these 'Find Your Me-Spot' events explained: 'We launched a national roadshow enabling women to escape from their hectic lifestyle for a few hours and enjoy quality me-time.'[26]

At the nights out, which were held all over the UK, women could choose from fashion workshops including 'What's hot and what's not – any excuse for new shoes!' and a 'Flirty something confidence class'.

The evenings were marketed by PR company Incredibull, which, in turn, was financed by Bayer Healthcare. They describe this project as a case study:

> 'The find your me spot' multi channel campaign targeted busy women in their 30s and 40s to think about their contraception choices. A combination of media relations, editorial partnerships, 13 city roadshows, digital content and celebrity endorsement encouraged women to find some 'me' time and focused on how to re-ignite their sex lives. The results? Extensive national, consumer and regional media coverage, with 86% of women who fedback at the roadshows feeling more aware of their contraceptive choices.'[27]

Indeed, Bayer Healthcare makes contraceptives, which explains why the evenings also offered 'contraception clinics'.

> 'Among the hectic chaos that dictates your day-to-day life, contraception may be the last thing on your mind. However, surely it's worth considering if it can transform other aspects of your lifestyle? There are a significant number of options available to women but do you know what they are? Did you know there are methods of contraception that you don't have to worry about for months, even years on end? Discreet yet intimate pods allowed guests to enjoy private consultations with experts in women's

health who helped them understand the options available. These were a great success with 86% of women feeling that they felt more confident and aware of their contraceptive options as a result of the consultation and 88% saying they will visit their GP/local Family Planning Association clinic as a result of the contraception consultation.'[26]

Contraceptive choice is a good thing. Women should have good, unbiased information about all the choices available to them. But is the best source of information an event run by a contraceptive manufacturer, a point that was not obvious in the media coverage of it? Is the best person to advise a woman someone working for the manufacturer – or someone independent and with access to full medical records with information about previous contraception use, problems, and other health factors that may have an impact?

PR presenting as information

Sleep well, Live well is the name of a website provided 'as a service to medicine' by Lundbeck Ltd. Lundbeck is a pharmaceutical company, though it is not obvious from the name if you don't already know.[28] 'Good quality sleep is essential for everyone' they say, and the site offers 'sleep facts' as well as a 'sleep test'. In a downloadable leaflet the role of melatonin is explained as something vital to sleep: 'As we age, our ability to produce melatonin naturally decreases. It is this decrease over time which may cause sleep problems and insomnia, the elderly are particularly vulnerable.'[29] The message is that sleep disorders are common but treatable: the gist is quite clear. See your GP if you can't sleep. Drugs to treat this can be prescribed.

The PR company paid to produce and maintain the site is quite clear that this is the aim. 'Sleep disorders are becoming increasingly prevalent, and their serious impacts needed to be recognised, diagnosed and treated by healthcare professionals in the same way as other diseases. Pharmaceutical company

Lundbeck developed Circadian – slow-release melatonin – to emulate the body's natural way of inducing sleepiness. Incredibull was engaged to develop a website, *Live well, sleep well,* to provide information and advice to the public and healthcare professionals, which included an interactive sleep test enabling sufferers to monitor their sleep patterns and present this information to their GP . . . The campaign has resulted in increased uptake from GPs and general raising of awareness of sleeplessness as a major issue.'[30]

As a GP, this is the kind of thing I hate. Patients coming to me with a printout showing poor sleep, the 'awareness' that they have a 'disease' and a request for a new treatment, such as melatonin, all presented as a fait accompli. The pressure is on me to comply and to sanction the treatment. I am pushed into defence; I have to supply the drawbacks, the hazards, the unknowns. The inference the pharmaceutical industry may draw is that I am indeed a Luddite, wanting to ensure that the newest treatments are kept away from my patients, or cautious of budgets, prescribing infuriatingly conservatively and generally neither listening nor caring.

In fact none of the above is true – I simply want evidence. I want people to get fair information about what might help them – and what might not. I prefer to be actively assisting people, not letting them down. This is the problem with most interventions that are being keenly promoted by their manufacturers. If it was clear that they worked well, they would be approved by organisations like NICE and SIGN. Doctors would be using them and be audited to ensure that they were. But if you don't have evidence, or it is not clear that an intervention does good, or if there are pros and cons, marketers don't want to know. In their world, if you can make patients keen on a treatment, and encourage them to go to their doctor to ask for it, what could be better?

When you read the evidence about melatonin for sleep problems in adults, it is neither universally positive nor clear. Let us take a meta-analysis, that is, a study looking at all the evidence available, not just the positive studies, on melatonin in adults with sleep problems. Published in 2005, in the *Journal of Internal Medicine*, it concluded that: 'There is evidence to suggest that melatonin is not effective in treating most primary sleep disorders with short term use (four weeks or less); however additional large scale randomised controlled trials are needed before firm conclusions can be drawn. There is some evidence to suggest that melatonin is effective in treating delayed sleep phase syndrome with short term use.'[31] In 2006 the *BMJ* published another meta-analysis, which concluded that: 'There is no evidence that melatonin is effective in treating secondary sleep disorders or sleep disorders accompanying sleep restriction, such as jet lag and shiftwork disorder.'[32]

The *Sleep well, Live well* website is aimed at any adult with any sleep problem. The aim of the website, as described by the PR company, was simply to increase 'awareness' and visits to GPs. But the evidence is that melatonin is not great at treating sleep problems. Better research needs to be done in order to sort out who, if anyone, would benefit most from using it. My duty as a doctor is to explain and recommend treatments fairly. Is a website written at the request of a drug company the best way to give patients that fair information?

Could you have chlamydia?

Thanks to PR campaign after PR campaign, the sexually transmitted disease chlamydia has become part of the modern lexicon. According to the operations director of Moo Moo Marketing: 'So many people still don't know how easy and painless it is to get screened for chlamydia. We are about normalising and naturalising the process through our peer outreach workers.'[33]

So, sexually transmitted infections can be uncomfortable, painful, distressing or even, in the case of HIV and hepatitis B and C, life threatening. Not treating chlamydia was presented as a risk to longer term fertility. Normalising testing may have hazards, especially if it comes with the impression that having sexual infections is a 'normal' risk. This may lead to changes in sexual behaviour that increase rather than decrease overall infection rates. In fact, the evidence for screening young people for chlamydia – that is, testing people for the infection who have no symptoms of it – has always been contentious, despite what the public has been told.

In 2003 the Department for Health in the UK set up the National Chlamydia Screening Programme, spending more than £150 million in the process. The National Audit Office (NAO) found, in 2009, that the scheme was recommended by 'an expert group appointed by the Chief Medical Officer; the programme was launched without generally agreed, robust data on the levels of chlamydia infection in the general population of the young people of England.'[34] Without even this knowledge, it would be difficult to know if a screening programme would be effective or not. We mustn't just embark on new programmes and tests because we can. We need evidence; we need to test our hypothesis. A systematic review from the *International Journal of Epidemiology* in 2009 concluded that:

'There is an absence of evidence supporting opportunistic chlamydia screening in the general population younger than 25 years, the most commonly recommended approach.'[35]

Successful chlamydia screening would have to take account of risk in sexual behaviour – becoming re-infected, or untreated people infecting treated ones. Yet it would be difficult to work out any negative consequences of screening from the effervescent effort put in to attract young people to 'pee in a pot' or even 'wee for a wii' – initiatives organised by PR company MPad, which was contracted to 'offer awareness' about chlamydia urine testing with the lure of winning gaming equipment. The director of the PR company said that they wanted to 'promote regular testing as part of a healthy lifestyle.'[36] Just as cholesterol is focused on as a relatively simple cardiovascular risk factor to modify, with less emphasis placed on diet and exercise, so chlamydia, easy to test for and treat, is used as a simplified way to give an impression of sexual healthcare and education. The NAO found that 40% of young people tested for chlamydia did not also receive information about either contraception or safer sex.[34] Chlamydia might have a quick test. But does selling that test, without proper, holistic care, constitute value for money – or even a good service?

Can we even be sure that the long-term consequences of chlamydia infection are as serious as stated by the people offering us the urine bottle? Do we even know exactly how common infertility is after chlamydia infection? The NAO also said: 'Due to uncertainties in the scientific evidence on chlamydia, the Department does not know how often infection leads to serious health problems and hence whether it is cost-effective to invest so much money into the problem.' In fact, by the time the NHS had spent millions on chlamydia tests and actually looked at the hazards of chlamydia infection, it changed its mind about which healthy, symptom-free people should be offered the test. Official guidance published by my local sexual health clinic in 2010 now says that: 'The risk of harm from chlamydia is lower than previously assumed . . . opportunistic testing in the absence of relevant clinical reasons should generally be avoided.'[37] And guidelines produced by the British Fertility Society in 2010 found that there was little proof (as the society put it, a 'paucity of solid evidence') about the long-term effects on fertility in both men and women who had previously had a chlamydia infection, despite what the screening programmes and the PR companies had said.[38]

We know there are hazards and dilemmas attached to screening. We know that the evidence for screening for chlamydia was not as clear cut as the PR campaigns claimed. So why was the NHS so keen to spend its limited cash on PR companies?

The answer is partly because of the targets set for local Primary Care Trusts (Health Boards in Scotland), who were required to reach thresholds of screening as part of their contract with the NHS. The targets were taken as indicators of a well run PCT. So what did we get? We got PR companies like 90TEN, contracted to advertise testing to young people in one part of England, organising an:

'. . . innovative, targeted and interactive Frisky not Risky campaign that took Chlamydia screening directly into schools and colleges, while supporting outreach teams to engage effectively young people in their environment. The dramatic uptake in screening propelled NHS Waltham Forest to third best PCT in the country and the only Outer NE London PCT to achieve the national Chlamydia screening target.'[39]

Was any of this actually useful? The NAO had its doubts. The medical evidence was patchy. As a GP, I want to know something else: what about unintended harms? Not just where cash could have been better spent. Could testing for chlamydia have changed behaviour so that the rates of other sexual infections rose? We don't know – we don't have the evidence. The over-enthusiastic selling of a quick and easy test failed to disclose the deeper uncertainties of testing: winning a wii would be scant compensation for suffering unintended harm.

12

Professionals in pay

'Need tips, quotes, professional advice on cosmetic surgery, anti-ageing and skin concerns? We represent one of the UK's most renowned cosmetic surgeons . . . he is much in demand for his well honed rejuvenation skills and is often described as a "true artist" by both his peers and those who have been treated by him.'[1]

Press releases touting for coverage – that one was for Mr Jan Stanek, a surgeon of Harley Street – are common.

A while ago I was talking to a slim teenager who told me that she was saving up in order to have liposuction to her thighs. They were fat, she said, and looked dreadful. I must have looked doubtful because she told me that she had a date for her operation and showed me where her legs were 'fat' and going to be operated upon. Her legs looked absolutely normal and slender to me.

This young woman had already seen a cosmetic surgeon who had told her that her thighs could be surgically slimmed. Who knows what fashion, catwalks, magazines or friends had influenced her. One study has shown that young people who watched reality TV with favourable coverage of cosmetic surgery were more likely to want to alter their own appearance.[2] Another US study, which reviewed the literature exploring the reasons why people sought cosmetic surgery, found that 'body image, teasing history and self-esteem were associated with motivational factors for those patients who elected to seek cosmetic surgery.[3] Surgery comes with risks; you may not end up looking like you wanted to, procedures can go wrong and anaesthetics come with a risk attached. Cosmetic surgery is not often available on the NHS. Instead, patients are treated in the private sector where they are customers, entitled to buy whatever a surgeon is willing to provide.

This is the end result of a competitive healthcare marketplace, with customers, not patients. Reams of UK and European clinics offer this kind of 'customer focused' service. In effect this often means that doctors will do whatever the person in front of them wants, whether or not they need it. Is this good for us?

People's reasons for asking for surgery may mean that they are less likely to benefit from it – or more likely to be harmed by it. A study of university students published in the journal *Body Image* examined a phenomenon described as 'appearance-based rejection sensitivity'. This is a measure of how likely a person is to feel excluded because of the way they look. For all that it sounds like a clinical diagnosis, appearance-based rejection sensitivity is a tendency that some people will have more than others. In other words, many people who are mentally and psychologically well can still have this background fear. What becomes a problem is that, as this study found, students who have more concern over their appearance have a higher risk of 'body dysmorphic disorder' – and are more likely to accept the idea of cosmetic surgery in the future.[4]

Body dysmorphic disorder (BDD) is, as its name suggests, more of a 'disorder'. It can occur in mild form, which has been described as 'imagined ugliness', when people believe that they are more unattractive than others find them. At the more severe end of the scale, some people become seriously depressed, obsessional in their beliefs, or even suicidal.

Several studies have been done to find out how common BDD is in people attending cosmetic surgery clinics. Between 5% and 15% of patients attending clinics have been found to have it; if you look for it in the general population the figure is about 0.7%.

The risk factors for BDD are shyness, childhood adversity, such as teasing or social isolation, and anxiety.[5] The treatment for the disorder is not cosmetic surgery but cognitive psychology. Yet how many patients attending one of the many cosmetic surgery chains of clinics are given a psychological assessment? Indeed, because these clinics exist outside the NHS, the doctors working there have no automatic ability to access patients' NHS medical records. This means that a customer can give an incomplete account of his or her 'problems', which cannot be automatically verified.

Here is one cosmetic surgery clinic describing vaginal surgery:

'Vaginal cosmetic surgery is becoming increasingly popular for women in the UK. Women undergo vaginal surgery for various reasons. Often it is because women are dissatisfied with their genital appearance or they would like to increase their sexual experience.

Opting for vaginal surgery can lead to an increase in confidence and self esteem and can often make women feel more attractive, helping them to recreate sexual excitement and rejuvenate their love lives.'[6]

Normally, women have a curve at the bone just above their genitals, the mons pubis. Yet this is portrayed by the same cosmetic centre as a problem: 'Pubic liposuction can greatly enhance the look of the pubic region making it more balanced and contoured.'

This cosmetic surgery runs opposite to what is normal and healthy for women. When we consider the reasons why people might seek cosmetic surgery, is it fair that doctors turn into mere providers of services wanted? Or would it not be better for doctors to be on the patient's side and to concede that just because cosmetic surgery is possible does not mean that it is in patients' best interests?

Most studies that have tried to examine outcomes of cosmetic surgery procedures have not included a control group.[7] So, for example, when one study reports[8] that breast enlargement can 'increase a patient's own self-assessment of attractiveness and self-confidence,' the researchers have not matched women who had the procedure with women who, at one point, wanted to have surgery but did not. People may consider surgery at one point in their life but reach a state of better confidence later on even if they didn't have a cosmetic operation. Some surgeons have been too fast to pinpoint surgery as the trigger for better lives when other explanations are also possible. Some clinics are too eager to operate. Here is one 'problem page' request from *More* magazine:

'I've always had an excess piece of skin hanging from one side of my vagina. It doesn't cause any medical problems but I feel really self-conscious about it so I'm thinking of getting it removed. Is it a safe procedure to have done?' *Paula, 25, Manchester.*

Cosmetic surgeon, Mr Alex Karidis says:

'Labiaplasty, or trimming of the excess or redundant skin or tissue of the labia minora area, is quite common. Although the excess tissue doesn't lead to any symptoms or pain, sometimes it can cause discomfort or embarrassment as it rubs against your clothing, or becomes visible through tight fitting clothing such as leggings. From a surgical perspective, trimming off the excess skin is straightforward and can actually be done under local anaesthetic. Recovery is usually 2-3 days.'[9]

I find this quite amazing. Women naturally have labia that are not symmetrical; that's what they are meant to look like. We create embarrassment where none should exist. Cosmetic operations may, in effect, simply alter normality.

In private practice, Karidis may be very cautious about doing these operations. But the glowing media coverage, with the unmistakable fingerprints of PR all over it, leads to wide acceptance of such procedures. Experts are pimped out to journalists looking to write stories about beauty; and of course some doctors who run private clinics will have an interest in keeping up demand. In the private, demand-led sector, there is no guarantee of an expert who would urge caution, or suggest that perhaps there are good psychological reasons not to operate. There are even publications such as *Facial Plastic Surgery Clinics of North America*, which run articles simply focusing on how to derive 'maximum buying power with your media project' . . . 'this article reveals these tips that are the most effective and includes information on the use of experts and other professional resources that help increase the likelihood of a successful outcome for a well-planned and executed media campaign.'[10] The product – cosmetic surgery – is primped and primed by doctors and their PR team, eyeing and playing the press. Who benefits most from these services? The doctor – or the customer?

Self-consciousness may not be best treated by surgery. Paying customers are sometimes served best by a surgeon who encourages the person before them to put away their credit card and think again. Doctors can't be salespeople – they have a code of ethics, and a responsibility to do the best for the patient in front of them. They are not allowed to hand over medical care like it was just another business transaction. Or are they?

The GP contract with the NHS

Most healthcare contacts in the UK happen within primary care. Primary care is the first contact with the NHS for most people. From there, people are cared for completely, with the doctors, nurses, physiotherapists, pharmacists or counsellors available for medical care, minor surgery or mental health problems. They can also be referred on to secondary care, in other words to hospital specialists. Secondary care will usually be able to manage whatever medical or surgical care is required, but will, for less common problems, sometimes refer on to tertiary care, which tends to be for very complex and rare problems requiring super-specialisation.

The very oldest GP records I can get my hands on are the 'Lloyd George' thick cardboard A5 envelopes, which are still found stuck in the back of our older patients' notes. Doctors then didn't go in for much verbosity, and there is just a hieroglyphic fountain pen abbreviation now and then. Some just state the treatment dispensed. Doctors treated the person in front of them for the problem they required assistance with. When the NHS was set up, GPs were kept in a 'double bind' to the NHS. They were not full NHS employees and were instead paid per item delivered. This consisted of payment of fees as listed in the 'Red Book'. Mainly, the payments were for things like childhood immunisations and minor surgery, as well as how many patients were on the practice list. In the mid-90s, practices could opt to be 'PMS' practices, where income could be, under the Personal Medical Services contract, based on the work done the year before and handled by the local authority rather than central government.

In 2004 there was a nationally agreed change between government and the British Medical Association, the medical trade union. This got rid of the old-style contracts and instead offered payments for hitting certain thresholds, or targets. Rather than being paid per immunisation or per prescription for contraception, practices are now paid once they hit thresholds. There are still some payments made for standard items, such as £56.20 per patient, per year on the practice list,[11] but for other items payment was set in bands for 'achievements'. There are more than a dozen in the cardiovascular category, ranging from the numbers of patients with controlled blood pressure to patients who have had heart attacks or strokes and whom the practice has placed on the standard preventive medication.[12] For someone with diabetes, the recording of their body mass index, treatment of high blood sugars, high blood pressure and cholesterol, together with annual flu vaccination, are all 'targets'.

There are also 'contract indicators' for well people who do not have heart disease or diabetes. There are 'obesity indicators', where practices gain income by producing a list of patients who are clinically obese. Practices are paid for 'additional services' like cervical screening and some immunisations. There are other payments too, such as recording the smoking status of patients as well as advising them to stop. There are thresholds for numbers of 'cardiovascular risk assessments' that have been perfomed on patients. GPs are to ask new patients for their ethnic origin.

Each one of these items generates points, which in turn generate income for the practice.

For me at least, this also generates discomfort. When a patient comes in to tell me about her depression, I am reminded that she is overdue for a smear and needs to have her smoking status recorded, courtesy of the practice computer system. In fact, the first thing I see when I call my patient's notes up on my computer are the tickboxes for the contract that haven't been filled in against my patient's name.

The generous explanation would be that the contract reminds me to offer complete holistic care. But from my side of the desk, however, I have ten minutes to find out about her mood, her job, her family, her home circumstances, her alcohol and drug use, her previous treatments, her preferences for treatment, her follow-up, and to ensure that she knows what to do in the meantime if she gets worse. I often like to provide written or other material. I also have to make sure she is not at high risk of harming herself, and act accordingly if she is. Even if that ten minutes were to expand to 20, I don't know if I could cover it all. People usually come in because there is something they want to discuss: this deserves attention. The government contract agenda pushes in front of the patient.

Another charitable explanation is that the contract is helping to bring evidence-based medicine to the front line of medical care. And isn't it evidence-based medicine that I've said, right from the start, is essential? We can't practise good healthcare without it. But evidence-based medicine simply provides us with knowledge; it does not tell us what to do with that knowledge.

So, for those 'cardiovascular risk assessments' – the money in the GP contract rests on getting the blood pressure down to 'acceptable'. There is nothing in the GP contract that emphasises the information the patient should get about the potential risks and benefits of the treatment. If there were, perhaps fewer people would struggle with side-effects that make their lives miserable and instead make informed choices that reflect their own values.

Some of the stipulations of the contract have very little evidence base at all. Collecting body mass index measurements from my patients, whether or not they ask for it, generates income to the practice. But I am at a loss to know what to do with the data. There is no evidence that this method of measurement results in healthier patients or more patients achieving weight loss. The evidence presented in the small print of the GP contract, as a supposedly evidence-based rationale, refers to the much-discussed rise in the number of obese people in the UK.[13] None of it refers to anything useful to do with this information (except if you include making the results available to the government.) And the possible harms of automatic weight measurement are blinked away in the fixation with contract points and the computer screen. How many patients with potentially serious symptoms are put off coming to their doctors for fear they will be told to step on the scales and told they are fat? We have no idea, but I know that these people exist, uncounted, because they tell me so.

The GP contract was a fundamental shift in doctors' practice. Instead of doctors being trusted by government to do their best for the patient in front of them, they were contracted to respond to a set of targets, agreed between trade union and government, which are a part of every consultation they do.

Take a patient who has depression, as described above. I could provide good clinical care – listen, make a diagnosis, discuss possible actions, make sure my patient was safe – but still fail under the measures of the contract. The contract just wants a questionnaire filled in, designed to grade depression as mild, moderate or severe.

This isn't a neutral act. If I am asking the patient to fill it in, or we fill it in together during the consultation, then there has to be something I'm not doing instead. Rather than the patient being given space to talk, our time is used for the form filling of political imperatives.

As we have seen, there is good evidence that the PHQ-9 questionnaire, which is approved for use in the GP contract – and which, incidentally, was developed by Pfizer (which makes several antidepressants) and made freely available by them[14] – is not good at diagnosing depression or its severity.[15] The GP contract stipulates that the same questionnaire has to be repeated at three months, despite there being no evidence that this is useful for the patient or treating doctor. There is no evidence that using these questionnaires will result in better quality treatment for the patient – and thankfully, the PHQ-9 was dropped from the GP contract in 2013.

This shift to contract-based care is important. It means that doctors are not just using their professional knowledge and judgment when they interact with patients; the income to the practice depends on carrying out the rules set out by the contract, so there is significant pressure on individual doctors to do these things even if they are disruptive or possibly useless. Financial incentives change what happens in primary care: after the GP contract in 1994, a steady rise in the uptake of cervical screening was demonstrated across England.[16]

What does this mean for doctors' professionalism?

13

Political patients

The inverse care law

So far, I have focused on the problems of well people when they become patients, through screening tests or questionnaires, cholesterols or blood pressure testing. I've also explained why I believe it's important that doctors act as professionals who can put aside self-interest and vested interests in order to serve patients well.

But what happens when we are sick? What happens when we have a pain, discover a lump or feel depressed?

Let us take a young man who has been feeling anxious and agitated. He lost his job six months ago, laid off as a driver for a firm that was going out of business. Let's call him Jack. He has been sleeping late and is using cannabis to help him sleep. He is behind with his rent and without any close family ties nearby. He becomes more anxious and depressed over a period of months, eating badly and drinking more alcohol. He eventually phones a helpline, and struggles to articulate what is happening to him. His financial, psychological, social and substance misuse problems are all contributing to his misery.

Jack is told to self-refer at a local mental health clinic. He is not sure where it is, or how to get there, but eventually he finds it and waits to be seen and assessed. After waiting half an hour he gets agitated and leaves. He tries again in a few weeks, when it is busy, and he is asked to phone to make an appointment. But the phone line is only open at certain times, which he struggles to remember, and when he does phone, he doesn't explain himself very well. He is given an appointment for a few weeks later. By this time he is using more alcohol and cannabis, in an attempt to self-treat his anxiety, and he sleeps in, wasting his appointment.

What would help? As a GP, I could help to begin to unwrap his problems and suggest ways to improve his situation. It could become clear that he is addicted to cannabis but his depressed mood means that he sees little point in trying to stop using it – he may tell me that it's the only coping mechanism he has.

I know that he would benefit from seeing a drugs and alcohol specialist nurse, skilled in helping patients to reduce or stop substance misuse. This approach would give him psychological counselling as well as monitoring and support.

But how does he get this help? The traditional way used to be a letter from me to the person I think he needs to see for help. Self-referral systems subvert this route. We now have these for primary mental health services, physiotherapy, podiatry and addiction care. Typically, patients have to phone in at specific times to arrange appointments. Often the first appointment is triage, and the second appointment is for assessment and possible treatment. This means the person needs a level of organisation and commitment to get treatment. But what if the illness reduces those abilities?

Self-referral systems for capable, relatively well, and articulate people are a different matter. They might be useful for people who can recognise their need for a particular service, know how to access it, and can then negotiate their way through it. But the less well, the less demanding, and the less aware of their 'rights' people are, the more difficult it is.

This is not a new phenomenon. The 'inverse care law' was first described by Julian Tudor Hart, a GP in Wales, in 1971 in the *Lancet*. He wrote:

'The availability of good medical care tends to vary inversely with the need for it within the population served. This inverse care law operates more completely where medical care is most exposed to market forces, and less so where such exposure is reduced.'[1]

Self-referral systems are relatively new in the NHS. They have been lauded as a way to empower patients and bypass obstructive doctors; the website NHS Choices says that this is useful for counselling, when people 'prefer not to talk to their GP'.[2] A self-referral system for physiotherapy is useful for 'empowering patients to self-manage their condition'.[3]

Leaving aside the semantics (self-management would, by definition, not involve a physiotherapist, just oneself), what hasn't been addressed is whether or not self-referral is good for those who may need treatments most. Indeed, most research into whether or not self-referral systems work has not examined potential harms. One possible exception was a review article published in the *British Journal of General Practice* in 2010.[4] It praised the 'Increasing Access to Psychological Therapies' (IAPT) programme, which was set up by the Department of Health supposedly to reduce waiting times for psychological therapies. The authors claimed that these systems did not just appeal to the 'worried well', but people with high levels of distress in need of care. Their view was that a 'self-referral route can be used to open

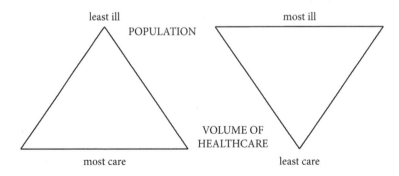

The inverse care law.

up pathways to care, enabling people to access services of their choice without having first to consult their GP', and one paper they cited in support of this was the pilot study for self-referrals, carried out in England and reported in 2009 in the journal *Behaviour Research and Therapy.*[5]

The pilot study was not a randomised trial, but an observational study. It was not designed to look at potential harms. Who did not get care because of this self-referral system? Who didn't manage to get through on the telephone, perhaps because of illness or distress? The pilot study researchers concluded, from comparing the depression questionnaires – such as the PHQ – that the service was useful and that 'opening up a service to self-referral was beneficial'. They even praised the: 'truly impressive level of throughput'. Throughput there may have been but was that useful to the most vulnerable patients who sought help? The authors found similar levels of distress in patients who self-referred and GP referrals. Yet as we have already seen, many people will complain about mental distress without having a mental illness. Questionnaires do not contextualise illness. And people who did not manage to get care for themselves were not filling in the forms.

GPs are regularly described as the 'gatekeepers to secondary care'. This can mean, effectively, rationing services; most problems will be dealt with within primary care and not referred on. Inappropriate NHS work, for example, cosmetic surgery, can be declined. But it also means triage, where urgency can be ascertained and addressed. It also means that a provisional diagnosis can be reached, and the best service to deal with the problem identified. Taking the first steps to sort out a mental health problem can be therapeutic in itself: a GP may be able to make suggestions that can be started immediately. Importantly, that person is then followed up. If a decision is made to refer someone for further treatment, and that person doesn't go for treatment, the GP is notified and is in a position to ask whether this means that the problem has got worse.

Throughput and good clinical care

The emphasis on 'throughput' is not surprising in a system that places such value on counting the numbers of people entering and exiting it. What about how good – how relevant and useful – the care was? The IAPT government report made play of the new 'skillmix': people who could come from a variety of backgrounds, not necessarily healthcare, and have a short training period before starting work in self-referral settings. These new posts effect changes on the rest of the primary care mental health team, which may include psychologists and psychiatric nurses. Essentially, it means that less 'severe' mental illness is dealt with by less trained personnel. Is this a good thing? One psychiatric nurse has written about the problems of making this distinction:

> 'Community psychiatric nurses in the United Kingdom are being repeatedly urged to focus their attention upon those with serious and enduring psychotic illnesses, and to withdraw from working with the 'worried well' in the primary health care setting. In view of this pressure, it is important to discover the role of the community psychiatric nurses' non-psychotic caseloads. . . these patients did not, in general, suffer from minor, self-limiting conditions. They typically had five years of contact with psychiatric services, and their psychiatric symptoms blighted their occupational, social and personal lives. Their condition caused significant carer burden, and there was frequently a risk of suicide.'[6]

Some people might like the idea of classing mild mental distress as 'stress' or 'anxiety' without an ongoing mental health diagnosis. It may be preferable for some people to have a less medical term for their distress and for it to be 'normalised'. Certainly, this is akin to what already happens in contemporary society – bookshops have shelves of books on how to treat low self-esteem, pressure at work or anxiety. Yet this low key approach isn't what people with severe or life-impairing problems may need. In the pilot study quoted on page 205, 'the service did not provide patients with a formal diagnosis'. When less generic mental health advice and more specific treatment are appropriate, a diagnosis is essential to enable better, tailored, treatment. Further, there are scant studies following up the long-term impact of such low-intensity interventions with patients, meaning that we have no data on whether this really does make a difference to even relatively well people in the longer term. It may even be that self-referral systems actually do the *opposite,* and medicalise mild problems rooted in life events or social issues that may have resolved themselves without a self-referral intervention.

So, do self-referral systems, and their inbuilt bias towards less severe disorders, work to the detriment of people with more severe mental health problems? Here is an extract from the *Royal College of Psychiatrists' Bulletin*:

> 'This has led to removal of consultant psychiatrists from assessment, diagnosis and treatment planning, but non medical staff have not been able to take over this role because they are not adequately trained. This has resulted in services that are not capable of offering psychiatric assessments and treatment.'

This sounds outrageous – a mental health service not capable of psychiatric diagnosis? The RCP article states:

> 'Attempts to improve psychosocial care for people with mental illness focus on non-psychological support. This has been at the expense of proper diagnostic assessment and prescription of treatment by psychiatrists aimed at treatment of specific disorders and recovery. . . [There is] a creeping devaluation of psychiatry which is caricatured as narrow, biological, reductionist, oppressive, discriminatory and stigmatising.'[7]

The same authors went on to describe how a liaison psychiatric worker was asked to assess a 'thin, withdrawn, dehydrated' woman after her GP had asked for a psychiatric opinion. The worker referred her to an eating disorders clinic. In fact the woman had a psychotic depression, diagnosed after the GP demanded a further opinion, and the woman required inpatient care with

ECT. Her treatment led to a complete recovery. There is no point in bickering about such anecdotal mistakes but this does illustrate that, while mental health systems may be cheaper to run with less well trained staff, we cannot expect less well trained staff to have the knowledge or skills of an experienced medical graduate.

When psychiatric hospital bed numbers started to fall in the 1990s, with the 'care in the community' policy, it was clear that many people had been institutionalised for decades and with no good reason. There was a shift to 'crisis teams' consisting of nurses or healthcare workers who visited people at home rather than admitting them to hospital. Again, this came partly in response to a perceived 'stigma' of psychiatric illness. However, round-the-clock, inpatient care remains the best treatment for some patients.

Mark, a person I interviewed for a newspaper article, is typical of many who say that getting inpatient care for severe illness can be very diffficult. 'I knew the signs' he said. 'You get to know your warning signs and I asked to go back to hospital. But they wouldn't have it. I ended up taking an overdose and being admitted to A&E – no hospital beds were saved.'

In fact, psychiatric bed numbers are now just above where they were in the 1850s.[8] The Royal College of Psychiatrists notes that independent surveys have found bed occupancy rates to be 100-140%.[9] This means that, rather than patients being cared for in a specialist psychiatric setting, wards are either overcrowded or patients are put on general wards instead. Additionally, with *New Roles for Psychiatrists*, published jointly by the NHS Modernisation Agency and the BMA in 2004,[10] psychiatrists were being moved out of direct patient care. Instead the report offered two models for the future:

'The director of care who is directly involved in determining care plans for all patients with a team that acts like a Personal Assistant, gathering information, triaging, and then doing the leg work...

The consultant who works with a team to establish a culture and possibly guidelines or protocols but then is brought in only when necessary with the team making and taking responsibility for many of the clinical decisions.'[10]

Compare this to the old way of looking after patients, based on 'firms', with small teams of doctors, nurses, psychologists and occupational therapists jointly caring for patients with the consultant psychiatrist taking overall responsibility. The old-style team would have had outpatient clinics to run as well as inpatients on the wards, and may also have had responsibility for day patients. Modern mental health care means that responsibility is more fluid. The government's 2007 *New Ways of Working in Mental Heath* report insists that: 'Many patients with uncomplicated conditions could be seen by less specialist staff working to protocols or trained in specific skills.' Yet it is only in retrospect that we can call the progress of an illness or treatment 'uncomplicated'. The report goes on to say that psychiatrists 'need great subtlety and understanding of group dynamics within teams and Trust clinical governance arrangements so that they can avoid accepting covert responsibility for the convenience of others rather than where appropriate.' It thus becomes less likely for a patient to see a psychiatrist.

A vexed issue for GPs in the UK is the problem not just with self-referral systems, but referrals made by GPs to mental health teams. The GP writes a letter of referral based on the assessment and the patient's preferences, together with a knowledge of the patient's history and social circumstances. The GP may ask for the patient to see a psychiatrist for specific advice on medication or diagnosis, or a cognitive therapist for specific treatment of, say, obsessive compulsive disorder. But that request may be overriden at a multidisciplinary meeting.

This may sometimes be useful: a GP may be unaware of a specific service that would be better. Yet the system is more frequently used to downgrade referrals. A patient who is shy or embarrassed about his depressive symptoms and their roots in his childhood may discuss with me why he would prefer to be seen one to one by a psychologist than in a group setting. But this discussion can be dismissed by a team that has never met the patient and doesn't have to answer to him. Additionally, a patient's care may now be routed through several different teams: the New

Onset Psychosis team, the Crisis team or the Community Adult Mental Health team. An unwell person, who may be paranoid, very anxious, suicidally depressed, psychotic or manic, is likely to prefer a doctor known to him to be in charge of his care, not another stranger.

This shattering of direct responsibility can be hard on primary care doctors like me, who are trying to work out where best to get advice for our patients and are having problems when requests for help are turned down. And it's even harder on patients.

Diagnosis by protocol is cheap but has hazards, as discussed earlier. When people call NHS Direct, or NHS24 in Scotland, they are asked a series of questions meant to direct them to the most appropriate care. This helpline has been staffed, as previously noted, by nurses as well as trained workers but the Department of Health has intimated that more basic workers, with just 60 hours of training, could be used, with only one trained nurse per 25 of them.[11] If you need simple advice or are not very unwell you are likely to have quite a good, quick service. But if you have a complex set of medical circumstances, you are more likely to have to wait for your turn to speak to a nurse, who may then in turn have to wait to speak to her supervisor or a doctor.

We already know that a huge number of people do not phone anyone for advice when they are sick, let alone the NHS. Every day, people with upset stomachs, a headache, indigestion, a touch of back pain or a cut to a finger sort themselves out with no help from anyone. Some people will ask at a pharmacy for advice; others will contact their GP, or indeed an NHS telephone service.

Until now, we have relied on patients themselves to choose where to go. Pharmacists have steered patients with significant symptoms towards GPs, and GPs have given patients diagnoses and advice about what treatment to take and what to do if symptoms get worse.

The Self Care Campaign was launched in 2010 and called its 'white paper' *Self Care: An Ethical Imperative*.[12] It claimed that a fifth of GP workload was related to minor ailments and this was a 'testament to an NHS addressing demand rather than need'. The campaign said that its 'key objective was to bring an end to the culture of dependency on the NHS for minor illness'.

It's curious, isn't it, that if you are well you will be contacted by the NHS to attend screening. But should you be unwell, you may be left to decide for yourself whether your constellation of symptoms should be described as 'minor' or not, and to sort yourself out.

In fact, the list of conditions that the campaign calls 'minor' includes acne, migraine and cough. Given that acne is often better treated with prescription antibiotics, that migraine needs a clear diagnosis and is usually better treated with specific medication, and that cough can represent many things from asthma to viral infections, pneumonia or cancer, it's difficult to say that these symptoms are ones that you shouldn't bother a doctor about.[12]

The Self Care Campaign was endorsed by various Royal Colleges, and advertised by the Proprietary Association of Great Britain (PAGB).[13] This association represents the manufacturers of over-the-counter (OTC) medicines and food supplements. On its website it tells us that the current value of the UK OTC market is £2.3 billion, with 973 million packs of medication purchased in 2010, the last available data. It also lists just about every multinational pharmaceutical company as a member.[12]

Let's put aside the reasonable question of why the Royal Colleges of Nursing and GPs were keen to work with this organisation, and concentrate on what the benefits might be for this vested interest.

The PAGB produced a report, 'Making the case for the self-care of minor ailments', in August 2009. It declared that 'The NHS cannot afford to spend £2 billion on minor ailments with expensive doctors dealing with conditions that people can cope with themselves and are already doing so.' Although it talks about 'significant savings', it is clear that the savings are from the cost to the NHS of prescriptions rather than savings for patients, who would be expected to buy OTC medication instead. It envisages the 'future picture' as: 'Confident consumer selects OTC (over the counter) medicine and makes pharmacist first port of call if symptoms persist.'[14]

I have vague ambitions of opening, one day, an evidence-

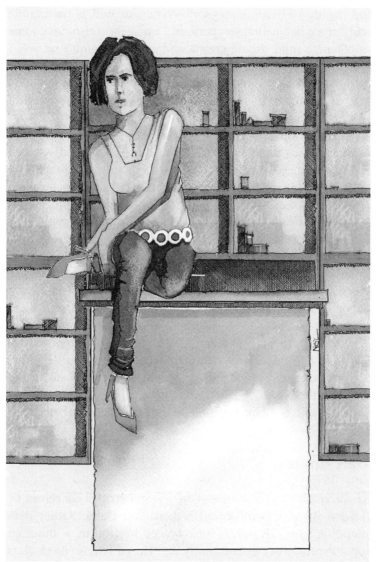

"I have vague ambitions of opening, one day, an evidence-based pharmacy."

based pharmacy. It will have many empty shelves. It will likely contain, for OTC use, paracetamol, aspirin, ibuprofen and possibly diclofenac. It will keep folic acid in stock, for pregnant and hoping-to-become pregnant women, as well as tranexamic acid, for women with heavy periods. I am likely to also stock some emollient, a mild steroid cream, and an antihistamine or two. I may stock a few other items that have some potential benefits, such as metal nit combs, but these would be likely to be sold only after discussion of the pros and cons. The remaining shelves will be happily empty.

Most pharmacies contain far, far, more. They have cough mixtures that claim treatment distinctions between dry, moist and tickly. They carry branded versions of anti-inflammatories, some in combination with codeine, more expensive than the plain generic sort. They have shelves of vitamins and food supplements, muscle sprays and various kinds of testing kits, as previously noted. There are also diet drinks, 'detox', homoeopathic remedies, chest rubs, as well as flu and HPV vaccinations. The products that would be in my evidence-based pharmacy are cheap, because they are out of patent and produced without branding and generically. Lots of stuff you see heaving on pharmacy shelves is not there because it has been evidence approved. Indeed, rereading that PAGB report, there is no mention of either the need for accurate diagnosis or evidence for treatment when it comes to self-care. Rather, the tone is about shifting people from the GP surgery to the pharmacy.

Is this shift good for patients – or the pharmaceutical industry?

Walk this way

An alternative to GP surgeries were Darzi centres conceived by Gordon Brown's health minister Lord Ara Darzi. Rather than attending your GP, people were invited to drop in, without an appointment. They opened early and closed late; some doctors felt they were new competitors to traditional GP surgeries. There was to be one in every local primary care trust area.[15] Many were run by private companies and the services they offered were very different from typical general practice. Most GP surgeries are staffed by doctors at various stages of their careers; there is usually a mix of experience. GPs are in the majority with nursing staff sharing some routine work in caring for people with some chronic diseases like asthma or diabetes. Darzi centres were different. The average staffing ratio was 1.2 nurses to every GP, with some centres being a 'nurse-led' service with a ratio of ten nurses to three doctors. Additionally, the doctors recruited to work in these clinics tended to be at the beginning of their careers.[16] Doctors complained that services that had been removed from their surgeries, such as physiotherapy and phlebotomy, due to a lack of resources, were to be reinstated at Darzi centres. A total of £250 million was spent on setting them up.[17]

Here's the paradox of patienthood again; these centres appeared to be best suited to people who were actually relatively well. Once again, resources were not being directed at those who were most unwell.

I'd prefer to quote you research showing the effect of Darzi centres on patient care. There is little: harms are rarely examined in policy-led changes to our health services. But take the response of a GP, writing in the *BMJ*:

'Our experience shows that even with good GP access many patients are using the walk in centre (WIC). We are a medium sized practice and have one of the highest ratings in our area (and well above the English average) for access to a GP within 48 hours. We see urgent cases on the day and seriously ill people without delay. We have a well established 'no quibble' policy of seeing children, whatever the problem, on the day. Yet every day several of our patients go to the walk in centre, many of them children. On each day there are unfilled urgent slots in our practice. My review of recent attendances by our patients shows they attended the WIC mainly for immediate access for minor self-limiting conditions. A review of this weeks' attendances shows colds, minor skin conditions, resolved upset tummies, minor muscle sprains, second opinion seeking. Patients were not prepared to wait even a short time to see one of our doctors – they were looking for instant access rather like when you pop into a shop for a pint of milk. . . . We are catering for 'wants' not 'needs'. In fact people didn't really want it but as it's there, and they have no idea of the cost, it seems they think they may as well use it.

As well as the waste of resources, the WIC model of care undermines the service we provide – because the WIC staff don't know our patients they can't provide continuing or comprehensive care and in some cases this has led to significant health risks for our patients or missed opportunities to deal with ongoing issues.'[18]

Darzi centres were expensive. Freedom of Information requests in 2009 revealed that patients who chose to register there generated an annual income of up to £560 each, far more than the payment made to ordinary GP surgeries.[19] With the expense and inefficiency of Darzi centres becoming clear, construction was halted by the Coalition administration in 2011, only for the private companies – and indeed, consortia of GPs setting out to profit from the tenders – to set forth a regulatory challenge to the government, saying 'this flies in the face of the Government's own commitment to take into account patient choice.'[18]

Choice is used as a justification to put resources where they are least needed. Once more, NHS money seems to focus on those who are well or almost well, with the truly unwell coming a distant second.

Referral management centres

When you consult with your GP about a medical problem, the ideal is that the two of you decide, together, what your concerns are and what to do about it. You may decide that a mole does not look quite like a mole should and decide it should be removed. You decide to book an appointment at a dermatology clinic. Or perhaps there is a problem with recurrent abdominal pain which you decide, together, merits an appointment with a gastroenterologist.

This kind of careful decision making is the staple diet of general practice. Doctors convey what they are concerned about diagnosing, and the limits of their certainty of it. Patients convey what they are worried about, what their symptoms are, and what investigations or treatment they would prefer or be willing to have.

This kind of consultation can be delicate and difficult. I do not want to alarm a person with what I may be worried they have: equally, I do not want to misinform or be dishonest. A person may have reasons to want a particular test or be fearful of another. It is the work of the consultation to find out about symptoms, family history, work issues, the impact on the home environment and the family, and to work out a plan that is acceptable on all these levels. It may be based in part on my knowledge of the patient, and whatever illnesses they or a partner or child has had. It will be guided by the knowledge of where we live and what services we have available. It will also be based on the undergraduate, postgraduate and continuing educational knowledge that I have.

And yet these careful, joint decisions may be entirely overridden by a paper-chasing process miles way. Referral management centres were set up in the mid-90s in order to 'monitor, direct and control referrals from primary care. Some also decide on the best treatment route for patients, which may involve redirecting referrals to other health professionals (eg a different hospital specialist, GP with a special interest or nurse specialist) or returning the referral to the GP to deal with in the practice'.[20]

Some of that might be quite good. Supposing, for example, that I am unaware that there is a specialist nurse dealing with the fixing and fitting of catheters to the bladder for someone needing them long term: this might be better dealt with by a nurse than a consultant urologist. But some of this redirection may be an additional time-wasting layer between doctors and getting the patient to the right person. GPs in one area of England found that 12% of their referrals were being rejected or diverted by the referral management centre.[21] In some areas private companies were used to run the referral management centres.[22]

This is obviously a major shift in the way in which GPs and patients interact with secondary care services. How is it justified?

The evidence on which referral management centres have been

based is not as clear as patients or doctors would like. Research about referrals is encapsulated in a Cochrane review, which was published in 2008. It said: 'There are a limited number of rigorous studies to base policy on. Active local educational interventions involving secondary care specialists and structured referral sheets are the only interventions shown to impact on referral rates based on current evidence.' Even the evidence that pre-structured referral forms, rather than the usual letter addressed to a clinic, were beneficial was only examined in certain well defined clinical areas: infertility, enlarged prostates and blood in the urine.[22] Yet only a minority of referrals deal with clear-cut problems such as these. Most problems do not fit into neat categories. How well can a referral management centre respond to a more difficult clinical problem? We don't have evidence to tell us that it's a good thing. As far back as 2006 a paper in the *BMJ* had concluded that 'evidence that the centres are effective is lacking, and costs are difficult to predict: assessment of referrals has the potential to introduce error and delay.'[23] It took until 2010 for healthcare thinktank the King's Fund to review the evidence and to tell us that these centres were 'failing to improve quality and deliver cost savings.'[24] The King's Fund is also keen to tell us that 'evidence shows that not all GP referrals into secondary care are clinically necessary, or require care to be provided within hospital settings.'[24]

When a GP refers a patient into secondary care, a decision has been made between patient and doctor. Evidence can and should guide us, but it is always flawed, never perfect, and will always come with uncertainties attached. Patients are entitled to make their own choices around evidence, and not to be forced into particular pathways or down a singular guideline.

Of course not all GP referrals into secondary care are necessary: good medical care is more subtle. The fictitious 'retrospectoscope', whereby we could predict the future diagnosis, would solve the problem of 'unnecessary' referrals but sadly it does not exist. So what referrals are worthwhile and useful?

The two-week wait

Screening tests are for people with no symptoms of disease and try to discover a disease process at an early stage. Most referrals that doctors make with patients are quite different. This means that people are suffering to a greater or lesser extent: pain, dizziness, coughing, the unknown nature of a lump. Diagnosis is necessary before effective treatment can be offered, or deemed unnecessary.

The 'two-week wait' was an entirely political, not clinical, invention. It was planned by the Labour government in 1998 in response to waiting times for routine outpatient appointments and a perception that Britain had poor cancer survival rates compared with other countries.[25] Previously, GPs like myself had three broad strands of referral. First, 'urgent', when there were worrying symptoms that could not wait for weeks. In these cases, I would send a fax or even try and speak to a doctor at the next relevant hospital clinic in order to ensure that care was planned appropriately. Then there were 'soon' referrals, which were for people without definitely deadly symptoms but who I was sufficiently concerned about. I wasn't happy with routine waits but equally I didn't think these people had to be seen very rapidly. Finally, the largest group was the 'routine' group. Probably different areas of the country had different systems but the shared distinction is this. If a woman had a craggy, hard, irregular lump in her breast, or a man had a bleeding, ulcerated rectal mass – strongly suspected cancers – I would be able to get care quickly from hospital clinics for that person. This was always the case.

Uncertainty is the watchword of general practice; rarely is it possible to be entirely sure about a diagnosis. Even in relatively common things, like advising about a urine infection, my advice will be to explain what I think the natural course of recovery will be, and ask my patient to return if anything untoward or unexpected occurs. When I refer someone to hospital for tests, it is often because I am uncertain about the cause of the person's symptoms. In many cases, serious disease will be in the list I am forming, Bayesian-style, as the consultation progresses. If I was able to predict with certainty which patients needed testing for underlying causes and which did not, I would save time, effort and money on my own and my patients' behalf. But this foresight is not possible. Research tells us so.

At medical school, doctors are taught about 'red flags'. These are symptoms that the doctor must attend to as a priority. Blood features prominently: blood in the urine, stool or sputum. Unexplained weight loss, a consistent feeling that there is a lump when you swallow – these are symptoms to which doctors are told to respond immediately; they are potentially cardinal symptoms of cancer.

And referring immediately is what I do, but how good is even such a 'red flag' in predicting cancer?

The General Practice Research Database is the world's largest computerised database of anonymised medical records held by GP surgeries. It collects data from 630 general practices, which amounts to about five million patients.[26] In 2009, the *BMJ* published a paper using this data looking at how useful 'red flags' were in picking up serious underlying disease such as lung or bowel cancer.[27]

Let's take coughing up blood, or haemoptysis. The researchers identified 4,812 patients with this 'red flag' symptom. Of these 297 were diagnosed with cancer of the lung. This means that only a small minority – about 6% – of people with a 'red flag' for lung cancer turned out to have lung cancer. Other problems that were diagnosed included infection, blood clots, bleeding disorders, heart problems, fluid on the lung, and chronic obstructive airways disease.

It's similar for other 'red flags'. Dysphagia, difficulty swallowing, was identified in 5,999 patients. Of these, 290 were diagnosed with cancer in the oesophagus or stomach up to three years later, meaning that 95.2% of people with this 'red flag' symptom did not have cancer. Instead, they had inflammation or narrowing of the gullet, a hiatus hernia, or an ulcer.

A similar story was described in a paper published in the US *Journal of the National Cancer Institute*, in 2010. This came during pressure from campaigns by cancer charities and institutions urging earlier diagnosis of ovarian cancer. Symptoms that were said to be suggestive of ovarian cancer were a feeling of abdominal bloating, a feeling of fullness, or urinary urgency or frequency. The study found that only 0.6% –1.1% of women with these symptoms ended up with a diagnosis of ovarian cancer.[28]

Clearly, most women with these symptoms don't have ovarian cancer. Another study published in the *British Journal of Obstetrics and Gynaecology* interviewed 124 women who had been referred to hospital with suspected ovarian cancer and declared in the abstract that 'ovarian cancer is not a silent killer', as it is often described.[29] The researchers found that women had been referred with a feeling of abdominal bloating, distention, loss of appetite or vaginal bleeding. However, these symptoms could also occur in women without ovarian cancer. In other words, the 'red flags' are, again, not exact and not terribly helpful when it comes to predicting who will be diagnosed with ovarian cancer. It is not the symptoms that are most helpful in making the diagnosis, it is the subsequent ultrasound scan, which is the beginning of the diagnostic tests.

The instigation of the 'two-week wait' policy was an attempt to triage. The intention was that GPs could sort out their referrals into likely cancer and not, and that this would lead to faster diagnosis of cancer and better survival rates. Yet, as I've described, the idea that a 'red flag' symptom will lead to a more exact cancer diagnosis is not what the evidence tells us. Certainly, we cannot ignore red flags, but nor can we rely on them for diagnosing cancer.

Here's another study looking at symptoms of bowel cancer. The same large GP database was used to look for people who had been diagnosed with this cancer, and matched them with controls who did not have bowel cancer. The researchers noticed that a minority of patients who ended up with a diagnosis of bowel cancer had one of the two 'red flag' symptoms, rectal bleeding or a change in bowel habit, at 15.6 and 11.2% respectively.[30] 'Most symptomatic colorectal cancers present with only a low-risk symptom,' they wrote. 'At least half . . . manifest low risk symptoms such as constipation or abdominal pain, and there is no intermediate test to identify those particularly likely to harbour cancer.' They pointed out that the diagnostic test in these circumstances is colonoscopy, which comes with a small risk of serious complications.

The bottom line is that the two-week wait rested on the premise that there was a magical formula for identifying cancer based on symptoms described to primary care doctors. But there is a problem: our beloved medical 'red flags' are not great at either predicting or excluding cancer. And of course, looking at symptoms purely from a cancer risk point of view diminishes other diseases still worth diagnosing and treating promptly – heart failure, for example, can have an outlook the same as many cancers.

The effects of the two-week wait were neither as hoped nor politically predicted. A meeting of the British Society of Gastroenterology produced evidence that 'the two week waiting standard is being met at the expense of a substantial increase in the waiting time for routine referrals, while not necessarily identifying treatable causes of cancer'. Two audits undertaken in district general hospitals had found that between half and two-thirds of cancer cases were found in the 'routine' rather than the 'urgent' waiting list.[31] A systematic review in 2009 confirmed this: 9.5% of patients referred under the two-week rule had bowel cancer, and 5% had stomach or oesophageal cancer. Two-thirds of patients who were diagnosed with bowel cancer were not referred urgently, but were mainly in the 'routine' list.[32]

This fits with the evidence: if you have 'red flag' or 'low risk' symptoms, it's hard to know which people will benefit most from being prioritised. One thing is sure; with such a burden of cancer in the apparently 'low risk' group, you have to be careful with 'routine' referrals. In 2005 the *British Journal of Cancer* reported on the effect of the two-week referral on lung cancer referrals.[33]

Lung cancer is a slightly different scenario in that many patients will be referred for further tests after a chest X-ray has been taken and found abnormal. The study assessed what happened to more than 1,000 referred patients, of whom 650 had lung cancer confirmed. They found that the two-week wait initiative changed the way patients were seen. The proportion of all urgent referrals seen within two weeks fell to 71%, having been 84% before the introduction of the two-week guidelines. Meanwhile, the proportion of all urgent referrals resulting in a diagnosis of cancer also fell, from 78% to 46% over the study period. The two-week wait did not change how early cancers were discovered. Instead, not only did waiting lists get longer but they concluded that: 'The two week wait scheme has so far failed to reduce waiting times for lung cancer.' The authors made it clear that routine referrals were neither useful nor fair. They simply deprioritised people. They concluded: 'Patients referred outside the 2-week wait are disadvantaged and thus practitioners would be wise to refer all their patients through the 2-week wait system.'

It would be tempting to wonder, as politicians are wont to do, if this is a problem that could be remedied by better education or training for GPs. But this does not deal with the immutable truth: it is hard to work out whose symptoms have a serious cause. The only thing that will help is to try to sort out timely further care for everyone with potentially serious symptoms. Prioritising one group over another based on symptoms that are incapable of acting as a fair judge of severity is not useful.

This wasn't just the case in bowel and lung cancers. In 2007, a *BMJ* paper concluded:

'The two week rule for breast cancer is failing patients. The number of cancers detected in the two week population is decreasing, and an unacceptable proportion is now being referred via the routine route.'[34]

This was what we already knew. In 2005, academics were stating the facts loud and clear, saying:

'Concerns have been raised over the often low yield of malignancy and the high proportion of malignancies still being diagnosed outside the two week wait system. There is, as yet, no evidence that the initiative impacts on survival.'[35]

Why didn't we test the two-week referral initiative before it was unleashed on the NHS, causing harm? Politics can't go before evidence. The two-week target was the one hospitals were told to meet, everyone else could go into an 18-week queue. By deprioritising people outside the two-week wait, we were making it harder, not easier, to diagnose cancers promptly. The comparison with screening is uncomfortable; well people with no symptoms are offered screening tests and investigations that are unlikely to save their lives. But if you have symptoms of disease, you may still get placed as a low priority. It would seem more ethical, more useful and more efficient to be less discriminating about which unwell people are seen promptly in hospital.

PART THREE

Making people better

14

What sort of patient?

When I graduated in 1994, the upper reaches of the austere hospital corridors were lined with dusty portraits of great physicians and surgeons, peering down with a censorious gaze. A fear of questioning 'higher' wisdom permeated the chill. Since then, physicians have lost their status as deities, thanks to the murderous intent of Harold Shipman and other widely reported 'medical scandals'. The loss of this remoteness and the new need for medical justification is a good thing. Doctors are human and patients are capable beings. Healthcare has stopped routinely bloodletting and frontal lobotomising, just because doctors believed it worked. Patients have learned to speak up, to interact online and to share information.

Concurrently, many healthcare charities and support groups have changed their focus. Many are no longer resources of financial aid and information for patients, and are instead challenging and campaigning lobby groups. Pharmaceutical companies have moved on from merely doling out pencils and post it notes to doctors via smartly dressed reps. Instead, pharma insinuates itself within patient groups, or offers 'education' to new prescribers, such as nurses and pharmacists. The message to doctors, too, has become more subtle, as pharma embeds itself within educational programmes, delivering its message in more clever ways than overt adverts ever could. Even NHS Direct has involved itself in a scheme in which AstraZeneca follows up patients on its asthma drug programme by telephone, with a pharmacy director of NHS Direct saying: 'NHS Direct is keen to run other patient support programmes with other pharmaceutical companies.'[1] An article in *PharmaTimes* in 2010 said: 'Pharmaceutical companies in Europe have long grappled with the paradox of an end-customer who is usually at arm's length and out of earshot. Public relations, media exposure and disease awareness campaigns can bridge this gap to some extent. But a more direct conduit to actual users of medicines has been through industry's relationships with patient organisations.'[2]

Is this what patients want? Do patients – or potential patients – want to be 'customers'? Being a medical customer entails all kinds of risks. It means being influenced by advertising, being lured into purchases through fear or fright, and invited to screening tests where the results might be indeterminate and of questionable significance. The customer's attention is competed for; the health consumer is reminded daily that there are health risks he or she is not sufficiently 'aware' of.

If the patients become customers, doctors become suppliers. Doctors would therefore work reactively, satisfying whatever fashion demands them to. Doctors should then proceed with whatever the customer wishes, whether it be a hazardous cosmetic procedure, a scaremongering genetic test or a prescription of evidence-free, side-effect-heavy, or hyped-up drugs. Profiteering from lucrative illnesses, or even making normality into illness, becomes the doctor's prerogative. Are people better served when doctors work without an ethical code and become technicians?

If so, it would work like this. No longer would anyone take any meaningful responsibility for our care. People and patients would have to shop around, and remember 'buyer beware'. People could be sick and frightened yet unable to trust anyone who offered treatment, because the 'treatment' could be useless, or more toxic than the illness. Care would be provided by people whose motivation was personal gain, not wellbeing; medical students would no longer be selected because they felt vocation or a desire to improve health services. Doctors would be free to earn fortunes by doing whatever they wanted and whatever people would pay for. Psychiatry and old age medicine, rehabilitation services and learning disability work in particular would flounder, since there is little scope for private practice or financial glory there. Health check-ups pandering to the basically well would thrive, seeing as they are based on customer demand, not evidence.

Or is there another way?

Expert patients

If you were to listen within the towers of the Department of Health, you would hear a clarion call to the 'expert patient'. This new title has been created and bestowed upon people who have chronic illnesses, who are called to attend a course, typically an hour a week for a set time, and led by a layperson. The Department of Health reports that most of us – 60% – have a chronic illness.[3] The course is offered to anyone with a 'chronic illness' from arthritis to seasonal affective disorder. But not all patients want to be intimately involved with their healthcare to the extent that it takes up even more of their time. The costs of being ill can include time taken to attend hospital and GP appointments, the ordering and collection of prescriptions, time off work when ill or recovering and, potentially, difficulty holding down a job. Chronic illness often has a disruptive effect on family life: we already know that many people are unpaid carers on many levels to family members and friends.

Again, this is the paradox of being a modern patient. The more likely you are to need help, or to benefit from medical care, the less easy it is to access it.

The 'Expert Patient Programme' (EPP) is run by the NHS, for patients, and boasts the slogan: 'Control your condition, don't let it control you' and offers 'the confidence, skills and knowledge to manage chronic health conditions such as arthritis, asthma, diabetes, heart disease and multiple sclerosis'.

One thing is unarguable: people should have access to good

information about health to help them make good decisions. People should also have the support they need. But the push is for patients to be involved in their healthcare to an extent previously unknown, with responsibility equal to that of doctors.

On one level that's valid. Patients, in the end, have to present themselves for treatment or take medication, not doctors. But should patients be responsible for ensuring that they get the best treatment with the fewest side-effects? How far should this responsibility stretch? Should patients be charged with searching the internet with the inference that better treatments are out there? This is what the EPP refers to as 'self-advocacy'.

Yet the more ill you are, the less able you are to do that homework. If I am so unwell that I cannot educate myself on the best treatment available, I want to know that someone else will do that for me. Why on earth should only the most motivated, literate and able people be further advantaged by their abilities to seek 'the best' in healthcare?

Doctors should ensure that their patients have the same good treatments regardless of their abilities to identify and find them. This is the hallmark of professionalism. Yet, as we have seen, unbiased advice and treatments can be difficult to find, for patients as well as doctors.

The EPP was evaluated by a team from the National Primary Care Research and Development Centre, which was closed in 2010.[4] In 2004, the centre published an evaluation of the EPP programme as it stood. Some of the comments are particularly illuminating. For example, on the naming of the programme, as noted by one of its administrators:

'Even the patients, for want of a better term, themselves have said that they don't like it because they say that just because they've got some sort of disability or disease doesn't mean that they're a patient. They don't see it as 'we're all prospective patients' they see themselves as being labelled again. And of course the GPs and the consultants don't like the 'expert' part of it because they don't see it in terms of that beautiful quote that was in the document, you know, which I think was something like 'my patients understand (their) disabilities better than I do'. They don't see it in those terms, they see it in a threatening 'I know what's best, you know nothing' kind of way.'[5]

The peculiar thing about the 'expert patient' nomenclature is the nonsense of it. Of course patients are the only ones who know how they are feeling and who are able to describe what is happening to them. They can be the only ones who know the level of uncertainty they are prepared to tolerate about their diagnosis, or which tests or treatments they want to have. But it is silly to start a competition between doctors and patients about who is the more 'expert' and in what. 'Patient' should perhaps describe the nature of a relationship with a doctor, rather than a person, and in the end, there is always going to be a difference between doctors' and patients' knowledge of a condition and ability to contextualise and place it in perspective. It is interesting to note that this competitive discord between doctors and those they are meant to serve has been introduced and propagated by politicians. We might ask why. Do we really want to set doctors and the people they have been trained to treat against each other?

In the meantime, we should ask if being an 'expert patient' does any good. One study suggests that those who go on these courses have a cost-effective rise in the quality of their lives. The measure used was the QALY (quality-adjusted life years), which was raised by the programme by a points score of 0.020.[6] A year of perfect health is scored at 1.0.[7] How meaningful, therefore, was this course in terms of people being better able to manage their condition? We are left a bit unsure. A Cochrane review published in 2009 looked at all the evidence available about self-management programmes led by laypeople, as the NHS scheme offers, and concluded that:

> 'These programmes may lead to small, short-term improvements in patients' confidence to manage their condition and perceptions of their own health. They also increased how often people took aerobic exercise. Whilst there were small improvements in pain, disability, fatigue and depression, the improvements were not

clinically important. The programmes did not improve quality of life, alter the number of times patients visited their doctor or reduce the amount of time spent in hospital.'[8]

The National Primary Care Research and Development Centre had also interviewed people who had taken part in an EPP course. It found that:

'. . . even those who report significant needs will sometimes portray themselves in a way that suggests positive social comparisons, which fit with a rationed and morally prescriptive and acceptable view of entitlement to NHS services. Such insights suggest that social comparisons in initiatives such as the EPP may be beneficial for some but exacerbate rather than alleviate health inequalities in long term condition management for others.'[9]

The bottom line: the most disabled gained less.

The EPP seems ill equipped to give greater resources to those who are struggling most with their condition or who are most disabled. Rather, it is the more articulate, well informed people, with time and energy to spare, who may be most likely to go along to these groups. Such people would probably have been able to get help for themselves anyway, even without the EPP. Indeed, as the National Primary Care Research and Development Centre found, this is exactly what happened.

'In the initial phase, the EPP courses drew in people already committed to self-managing and who tended to be white, middle class and well educated . . . if those who stand to benefit most from learning self-management skills (in particular people from ethnic minority groups and areas of high deprivation) are disinclined to participate, then one disadvantage would be to increase inequalities.'[10]

If a person does not go on an EPP course, does that mean that they are less expert than those who do?

The EPP is not serving the sickest patients well.

Self-management and sharing knowledge

Part of my dismay over the EPP involves the standardisation and lack of personalisation in the courses. Knowledge and resources are removed from the personal and confidential nature of a one-to-one consultation and put into a group setting. The courses, which have now seen the attendance of more than 80,000 people in the UK,[11] also move away from the natural way in which people with the same illnesses have traditionally shared information and support.

Giving people enough information about their condition and what they should do about it is ingrained in good medical practice. Indeed, the General Medical Council (GMC) makes it clear that doctors should 'support patients in caring for themselves to improve and maintain their health'.[12] That way, if discussing options for treating depression, I should ensure my patient knows what to expect and what to do if things get worse, to choose medication if required and what side-effects to anticipate, and how to deal with them. I'd also hope to suggest some decent books or websites, or phone numbers for extra support, as suitable. This personalised information is at the heart of consultations. Without this kind of discussion, the consultation will not bloom. I am sure I fail in this often – but dealing with chronic disease in general practice is seldom a one-off, but a recurrent relationship, where revisiting and elaborating can take place. A ten-minute consultation is hardly enough for most of this but it is a start. If a patient has asthma, for example, I would ensure he is also in touch with our practice nurse, who can provide follow-up education on, for example, warning signs of a relapse, and changes that can be made to medication. If a person has chronic bronchitis, we want to reduce exacerbations in the future: this may involve ensuring that the person has a supply of steroids at home, or is working on an exercise programme to improve lung function. These actions are nothing exceptional – just normal parts of good medical practice, when the patient and the doctor can agree on the best plans for that individual person.

The EPP is different. Traditionally, local groups, usually

run by nurses or doctors in tandem with patient groups, have ensured that newly diagnosed people as well as people in the longer term have information, tips and knowledge. Diabetes or epilepsy groups in particular have worked well, having been able to discuss specific problems with the local service or meet with one of the doctors to discuss the value of a new treatment. Local people had ownership of the agenda and these groups continued over months and years. The EPP, on the other hand, is scripted, and can be run by volunteer laypeople who may not have the same condition as the people on the course.

Giving information about illness and disease has been an essential part of medical care ever since doctors had information to impart. Doctors absolutely have to share that knowledge in a way that is relevant and useful for patients. The EPP is only for those who wish to attend – automatically, only the most motivated will get on the course. Is good information and personalised care not the aim of normal, routine, general practice?

In the meantime, the stuff that really would help patients become co-collaborators with doctors is absent from the EPP. Patients are left to the wilds of the media for information about new treatments without being given good advice about how to handle the claims that are made. It would be possible to show people with long-term conditions how to react to the latest 'discovery' reported in the press, but instead they get advice about healthy eating, which is already easily available from NHS resources. The EPP is guilty of providing simple customer fluff rather than addressing deeper patient needs; relaxation techniques and deep breathing exercises could have been learned at any number of local venues already.

No decision about me, without me: sense or spin?

This is only the beginning of the definition of the medical customer. In 2010 health secretary Andrew Lansley wrote the White Paper 'Equity and Excellence: Liberating the NHS', which promised: 'Patients will get more choice and control, backed by an information revolution, so that services are more responsive to patients and designed around them, rather than patients having to fit around services. The principle will be 'no decision about me, without me'. Under the new plans, patients will be able to choose which GP practice they register with, regardless of where they live, and choose between consultant-led teams. More comprehensive and transparent information, such as patients' own ratings, will help them make these choices together with healthcare professionals.'[13]

One way to work out if a statement is silly or not is to work out if the opposite is contestable. For example, if someone is 'against cancer' I contest that this is nonsense, because it would be daft to be 'for cancer'. So if it is really a breakthrough to consider that there should be 'no decision about me, without me', the opposite should be contestable. Since the opposite – forcing people to do things and allowing them no say in the matter – is ludicrous, I contend that 'no decision about me, without me' is slick, meaningless spin. Doctors do, rarely, have to become involved in going against the will of patients – for example, reporting a concern about child abuse or detaining a mentally very unwell person in hospital. For these, there are specific laws and specially trained social workers, not doctors, making the final decisions. Elsewhere, it has always been unethical for doctors to act against the will of the patient. This principle has endured past numerous governments and should not change even if party politics do. What would happen if a future government ordered doctors to force patients to take tests they didn't want? Doctors should never accept this kind of instruction. Medical ethics needs separation from transient political will.

Instead we have a political drive for patients to make decisions – except that these might not be the decisions we should be prioritising. Again, the political agenda supports the patient paradox: the less ill you are, the more care you get. If you are basically well and want to shop around for your hip replacement, you can go online and do so. If you are one of the estimated 9.2 million UK adults who the Office for National Statistics estimated, in 2010, had never used the internet[14] then you are automatically going to find it harder to do this. Even with internet access, we may not have the time or capacity to take on this type of responsibility. If we are very sick – seriously mentally unwell, in a great deal of pain, or if our attention is being diverted by distress or fear – it is rather unfair to expect us to take on the feat of finding the best care for ourselves.

Take Meg Gaines, a criminal defence lawyer in the US. She found that she was expected to make choices for herself when she was very unwell with ovarian cancer.

> 'The doctor then recited what has become the maddening litany of medical correctness: "We're in the outer regions of medical knowledge", he said, "and none of us knows what you should do. So you have to make the decision, based on your values." Ms Gaines, bald, tumour ridden and exhausted from chemotherapy, was reeling. "I'm not a doctor!" she shouted. "I'm a criminal defence lawyer! How am I supposed to know?" This is the blessing and burden of the modern patient. A generation ago, patients argued for more information, more choice and more say about treatment. To a great extent, that is exactly what they have received: a superabundance of information, often several treatment options and the right to choose among them. As this new responsibility dawns on patients, some embrace it with a sense of pride and furious determination. But many find the job of being a modern patient, with its slog through medical uncertainty, to be lonely, frightening, and overwhelming.'[15]

This is not an argument against information being freely available to patients; all clinical research should be made available to anyone who wants to look at it, free of charge. Nor do I think that doctors should take decision making out of patients' hands. Instead, it is a professional ethic to ensure that, as the GMC says: 'Relationships based on openness, trust and good communication will enable you to work in partnership with your patients to address their individual needs.'[16]

Just as medical omnipotence is dangerous, so too is onerous responsibility placed on patients. The inference the politicians make is that you should be actively involved in achieving the best care for yourself. Customers are to seek out medical information and assess it. The doctor, acquiescing to demand, fails to offer advice, direction or opinion. Health 'consumers', in the end, are responsible for themselves.

This philosophy disregards medical ethics and professionalism. Of course patients are responsible, at least in part, for many decisions made in all kinds of ways – how much alcohol to drink, how much exercise to take. The White Paper instead stated that there should be: 'a presumption that all patients will have greater choice and control over care and treatment, choice of any willing provider wherever relevant and choice of treatment and healthcare provider becoming the reality.'[17] The intention is that people should shop around and satisfy themselves that they are getting the best care possible.

The 'choices' that politicians set down are, once again, only of use to people who are pretty well to start off with. Let's see: via a hugely expensive system called 'Choose and Book', rolled out by the previous Labour government from 2005, patients were to be offered a choice of hospitals. In the NHS in which I trained, if you wanted your operation done, say, near family members to help with convalescence, then it was already possible to do this. So a lady, living on her own, and her daughter working full time and 400 miles away, might want to have her hip replacement done close to the daughter's home, where she could stay to convalesce. At any point in the past all I, as a GP, had to do, was to contact the appropriate hospital to make the arrangements. There was no infrastructure of internal NHS finance to bear down on humane common sense. Such requests were uncommon, but perfectly possible. This flexible, user-friendly approach has gradually been replaced by internal markets and competition between hospital trusts.

To reinstate the possibility of such choices, Choose and Book was introduced to general practices in 2004. This was not run on principles of co-operation, however, but of stick and carrot finance. Payments were made to GPs to complete referrals in this way, and we were incentivised to do so by more than £100 million over three years.[18] Doctors hated it, saying that it was time-consuming, and the system, devoid of a human interface, often sent patients to the wrong specialist. One cardiologist said 'This new system has introduced fault-lines into the patient journey that we have no control over. It's delaying treatment and making doctors' lives a misery. It is deeply depressing and we loathe it.'[19] Its projected costs were more than £200 million.[20] Before Choose and Book, consultants simply 'vetted' referrals from GPs, ensuring they agreed about the urgency of the request and the clinic the patients were sent to. This kind of sensible process became impossible as the computerised system was unable to think and adapt to new information. There was no Bayesian ability to make exceptions or override bad data. How, exactly, do the sickest patients benefit? They don't.

Being a doctor or a patient in a system that prioritises a sexed-up computer system over consistent and decent care for everyone isn't healthy. The definition of a competitive marketplace is that there are always going to be losers.

Rate my doctor

So how should newly 'empowered' patients make decisions about where to be treated? There is no teaching about evidence in the EPP, or information about how to judge raw statistics. Instead, politicians have pushed the idea that patients can review doctors either on the NHS Choices website, or other similar sites, in the same way as hotels are rated on travel review websites. Ben Bradshaw, health minister in 2008, said: 'I would never think of going on holiday without cross-referencing at least two guide books and using Trip Advisor. We need to do something similar for the modern generation in healthcare.'[21]

Does this benefit patients? Does using other people's ratings of doctors get patients better care? And does it help doctors to improve the care they give to patients?

We lack evidence that all this effort produces anything useful. Asking around a local area for a good GP practice has the advantage of ensuring that the people whose views you seek are real. I can choose whose opinions I trust; a friend is trusted, a stranger may not be. An online rating that puts someone off a certain GP practice may have been written by a person who has been (rightly) refused extended prescriptions for temazepam or someone who is unhappy at being told that he is now fit to work and cannot be certified sick. Asking a real person will let me know that the wait to see a popular doctor is worth it: if he runs late it's because he takes the time to sort out a patient's problem, not because he is drinking coffee and having a fly cigarette out the back. When in a waiting room myself, I overheard two gentlemen dismiss another's complaint that the doctor was running late: 'Aye,' they said. 'It's because he takes his time over you.' The problem with relying on people to go online to type a rating is that it is likely to generate responses that are either very good or very bad. We cannot be sure that we can trust the results.

This is important. Any serious study that wanted to demonstrate the effect of this scheme on people's decision making would have to try to collect fair data to start with. So, for example, in my surgery, every year, each doctor asks 50 patients for their views on their doctor and the practice. This means that the results belong to real people, and represent broad views. Should the government be recommending that people choose doctors based on data that may be incomplete or biased?

The other problem is for doctors. If I have a negative online review, what should I do? One complaint currently on NHS Choices is that someone had a bruise after having blood taken. Another complaint says that there was a failed diagnosis. But what happens next? I would count a bruise as a minor, expected and temporary issue, not even a problem. A missed diagnosis could be fatal. These complaints are accorded the same significance online. I would want to be able to find out what went wrong and why, and to rectify this, but online there is no trace of how to do so, or even how to find out if the complaints are unreasonable or a sign of serious problems within my workplace.

If a comment had come straight to the surgery from the patient, there would be a hope of improvement. I could quickly review the problem, discuss it with colleagues and if needs be, act quickly, as well as communicate back to the patient. Instead, patients are being encouraged by politicians not to interact directly with their local practice, but to go online and behave like commercial customers. We in small general practices do not have PR departments or media campaigns. We don't spend public money to operate like a corporate sales team, attracting and enticing customers. Neither should we; healthcare suffers when it is oversold, whether by doctors, patient groups, quick slogans or pharmaceutical companies. When patients are relegated to purchaser status, all they have is buying power and this makes them susceptible to the problems of sexed-up medicine in all its devious forms. The skill of sharing clinical uncertainty and medical unknowns is washed away in a wave of publicity messages and hard sells.

NHS doctors should be offering something better – their professionalism. Patients should certainly be asked for their views about how NHS services should be made better but this should help all patients, not just those able to look up reviews and take their healthcare elsewhere. Otherwise we simply cater for the healthiest and weathiest, and neglect everyone else. Choice is not necessarily meaningful or useful.

15

Not more information,
better information

Good choices need good information. So we need easy access to
results of large, randomised controlled trials (RCTs), free from
bias, with useful outcomes and long-term data, and fair estimates
of benefit or risk. With good information, choice is easier.

In reality, good information is scarce. We have thousands
of unanswered questions about what we are currently doing,
never mind what we aren't yet doing – just look at the DUETs
database (UK Database of Uncertainties about the Effects of
Treatments), which stores the hundreds of questions being
asked about the uncertainties of medical interventions.[1] We have
massive problems with getting good data of relevance to patients.
Drug or other treatments that don't work are far less sexy to
researchers and medical journals than drugs or treatments that
do work. The end result is that fewer negative results appear in
journals.[2] This generates a climate where we have more positive
information about treatments than fair information. And there
is nothing (apart from ethical considerations, naturally) to stop
pharmaceutical companies burying data they don't like the look
of and, as we have seen, they frequently have.

Then we have clinical trials themselves, which do not always
contain fair representations of the people the drugs are eventually

prescribed for. Statin drug trials, for example, have been made up mainly of men – 90% – and mainly middle aged, rather than older populations.[3] Many ethnic groups are underrepresented in cancer trials, with concerns raised about declining numbers of black people tending to enrol.[4] Clinical trials are keen to eliminate as much variation between participants as possible. This means that many people taking medication for multiple other conditions are excluded. So although the trial might be better by design, there will be question marks about how well the results will apply to the 'real world' patients outside of trial conditions. We also know that even interventions that are widely accepted as being good and are standard practice don't always help – such as a one-off dose of steroid for childhood croup, which helps only about one in five children to get better quicker.[5] We have already examined the small chance of benefit from taking a statin or blood pressure medication and the different ways of expressing that gain that could be used to persuade or dissuade us from taking it.

It seems that the more sellable a health problem is and the more sexed-up the proposed treatments, the worse we are informed about it. For example, the entire month of October is devoted to 'breast cancer awareness'. But we know that women underestimate the average age of being diagnosed with breast cancer, overestimate their risk of dying of it, and overestimate their risks of getting it.[6] The young women who often appear on breast cancer 'awareness' posters probably don't help.

What happens if you spend time and effort getting better information to patients? If men are given high-quality, unbiased information about the PSA test for prostate screening, fewer men want the test.[7]

But the idea of allowing people to make up their own minds about what tests or treatments to have has not been universally welcomed. Decision aids – information packs on paper and DVD – have been created and tested to find out what effect they have on people offered bowel cancer screening. The effect is pretty clear: better information means fewer people opt for screening.[8] A psychologist, responsible for research into helping people make decisions about screening, wrote in an editorial in the journal

Evidence-Based Nursing that this effect was 'disturbing'.[9] Another psychologist noted that while people who had used the decision aid were better informed about bowel cancer screening, the uptake of it might be reduced because of this better information. He said:

'A more appropriate framework in this context might be to structure the facts with reference to evidence on how to improve understanding of the disease, test, and treatment and to facilitate adherence with testing – that is, a policy of informed uptake rather than informed decision making.'[10]

In other words, change the information patients are given in order to get the result that you 'want'. The psychologist author was concerned by 'paradoxical findings that adults who received the decision aid were more informed and had positive attitudes to bowel cancer screening but were less likely to have faecal occult blood testing'. Why the paradox? This is true 'patient choice' – allowing people genuinely to make their own minds up about what screening to have. The conclusion of this psychologist speaks of a reversion to the dark days of medicine, when meek patients were told what was good for them to swallow.

Instead of celebrating a decision aid that got better information to people who could act as autonomous adults, we have healthcare professionals telling us that we should have our arms twisted instead.

Somewhere the fundamentals of medical ethics have been lost. Citizens and patients should know the truth about screening tests as well as treatment risks; and we should be free to choose, not coerced into one course of action. Some people might be most pleased to have their bowel cancer screening, others will decide that the chances of benefit are not worth the risk of false positives. Treating people as capable individuals is part of normal professional ethics and doctors should not just allow but encourage people to make decent decisions for themselves.

Forget the EPP. Screening choices are the kinds of decisions that patients should really be thinking about.

Stop screening, start living?

What would happen if we didn't take up every screening test on offer? In the developed world, where our life expectancy is increasing, and where we live healthier, better educated lives with opportunities to eat well, travel well, communicate more easily and reproduce safely, we are sold numerous interventions to improve our health, from those whole body CT scans to cholesterol checks. Yet, as we have seen, their benefits are far more limited than we might have been led to believe.

Life expectancy for children born in the US, a country in love with every health check going, is 75.1 for boys and 80.2 for girls.[11] In the UK, we expect boys born now to reach 78.2 years and girls 82.3.[12] We are living longer than a country that spends – or wastes – more money on healthcare. What about the way we spend those years? More health screening may mean that we spend a good portion of our lives being tested for diseases we were never going to get, or enduring treatments that were never going to change when or how we died.

Men having prostate screening may go on to have a biopsy that shows no evidence of cancer. You might think they should feel relief and sleep easy. In fact, men in this group are reported to worry more about prostate cancer compared with a control group of men who had a normal PSA test.[13] A false alarm has consequences; more tests can cause more anxiety, even if the results are normal. From the point of view of an ordinary GP, anxiety about health screening results is common, and false positives only make this worse. But when we tell women to 'renew travel card/book haircut/go for screening test/buy cinema tickets', as the NHS information leaflet on cervical screening does,[14] it hardly imbues the sense that this is a decision of gravity. Indeed, the only mention of an adverse outcome is right at the back:

'What would happen if I did not choose the test?. . .You can choose whether to have a screening test. If you are unsure about having the test, you can speak to your doctor or nurse, or visit www.nhs24.com/cervicalscreening for more information. It is important that you understand the reasons for screening, and the possible outcomes if you choose not to have a screening test.'

With this kind of stern warning, the risks of not having the test take precedence over the risks of having it. Many GP surgeries, so alarmed at the prospect of being blamed for not detecting cervical problems early, ask women to sign forms confirming that they understand the 'risk' of opting out. Yet there is no similar formal process for *consent*. The balance is skewed. We are treated like sheep in need of firm handling.

So what would happen if we cut down the amount of screening we did?

Take an overweight, chain-smoking and sedentary man in his fifties who is worried about a cholesterol of 6. From a doctor's point of view, it is easier to prescribe pills to reduce the cholesterol level rather than to start the hard process of how to reduce cardiovascular (and cancer, and dementia) risks by losing weight, stopping smoking and exercising well. Or take a young woman, who has read that she is 'low risk – not no risk' of developing cervical cancer. She is also afraid of the cervical smear. Full information might enable her to choose whether to take part or not, and if she takes part, and the result is abnormal, she will already know that a borderline smear result does not mean cancer is very likely. A pregnant woman might decide not to have ultrasound screening for fetal abnormalities, because she has information to tell her that she is low risk, and would not, in any case, want an abortion.

This proper treatment of patients as competent adults may have positive effects. Without cholesterol and its medication to distract us, we can concentrate on bigger, more holistic risks to health. Giving women decent information about screening allows doctors to stand by their professional standards, and treat women as adults who don't need a paternalistic NHS to make choices for them. So the pregnant woman is spared uncertainty about a scanning abnormality which was, in any event, non-specific, and baby was fine in the end. The young woman afraid of cervical smears is given information that allows her to make judgments and keeps her in control of what happens to her body. The obese, sedentary man considers that a cholesterol level will respond to weight loss and exercise, which, together with stopping smoking, will make the biggest impact on his quality and quantity of life to come.

The possibility exists that the harms of screening erode the marginal improvement on quantity of life they generate. Screening may simply make us sicker, overdiagnosed and overly concerned about inconsequential cholesterols, PSAs, and 'cells of uncertain significance' at cervical screening.

The parting of politics and health

Many of the problems that people are landed with in screening have their roots in politics. I am not thinking of any particular party; each has sought to control the NHS in a way that allows it maximum election-time leverage.

So we had Choose and Book, which was meant to give patients 'choice' about where to have treatments – except that it cost a fortune and patients didn't want it. We had breast screening, which Edwina Currie admitted was good for votes, despite the uncertainties about the evidence. We had 'well person' checks introduced by vote-seeking politicians, not because evidence said they would be useful but because opinion polls suggested they'd be popular. The NHS is tethered to the Department of Health. There is no holding chamber for daft ideas or committee for evidence through which all public spending must pass. NICE, which was established to assess whether treatments were useful and cost-effective was one good political creation, but has had wavering political support.[15]

Fundamentally, the NHS provides the healthcare we need, free of charge. However, 'need' is an outmoded concept in a society where most facilities are provided on the basis of who shouts loudest. But need is what our health services should be based on: it makes no sense that someone, say, in great pain and with a bad fracture of the arm, is put to the back of the queue behind someone who has a mild itchy rash. In healthcare, prioritising based on need is fair. It might be nice if we had enough healthcare staff permanently on duty to see anyone who wished to be seen within seconds, but a tax-funded NHS remains affordable because it triages the urgent from the routine.

Politics is distinct from the scientific process. Good science starts with the acceptance that we don't know the answer to a problem. Experiments are designed to reveal that answer; the generated evidence is questioned and firmed up and repeated, and if the results hold, the results are implemented. Politicians work in a different way: theory drives action. This is not to dismiss politics, but when we try to bend science and medical research to political will, it will not go. We end up with dead-end policies that weren't needed in the NHS and have wasted time and money. So for example, the National Audit Office noted that despite £2.7 billion being spent on electronic patient records, the scheme was not helping clinicians and 'does not represent value for money.'[16]

There is more. Launched in two waves over 2003 and 2005, independent sector treatment centres (ISTCs) were built in order to shorten waiting lists for surgical procedures such as hip replacements and cataract removal, and radiological investigations like MRI. These centres cost more than £5 billion and 23,000 NHS beds were closed in anticipation of their success.[17] They operated external to the NHS, treating patients referred to them. If there were complications or problems then patients were dealt with back in the NHS. How good was their care? What data did we have that showed that ISTCs were as good as the NHS? In a report to the Department of Health, the National Centre for Health Outcomes Development analysed the outcome data provided by ISTCs and said in 2005 that: 'We have no way of judging the accuracy of the data submitted.'[18] The then president of the Royal College of Surgeons, the late Hugh Phillips, noted that the ISTCs would often fly surgeons in from abroad to do the operations, who did not use the same type of hip replacements as NHS surgeons, selecting other types at odds with standard practice. 'It was not good enough for a surgeon to fly in from France and do five hips in a weekend only to have them "falling to bits" later.'[19] Similarly, ophthalmologists highlighted the problems with patients having cataract surgery in ISTCs: 'Mobile units which by definition will not be able to provide continuity of care for their patients. Patients with complications such as endophthalmitis or dropped nuclei will in effect be handed over to local departments to be "sorted out".' Take or pay contracts were given to ISTCs, which meant that they were paid regardless of how many operations were actually done. The private sector was given contracts even in areas where there was no need for more capacity.[20]

I recall exactly the same problem when I was a lowly resident: the arrival into the NHS of a sick patient from the private sector. Suddenly the patient is deemed too sick for the private hospital to care for, whether because of the need for more, or specialist nurses, or intensive care. This is simply a consequence of being a customer. The seller can terminate the contract.

Again the paradox: the least sick get the most attention. ISTCs were intended to take the routine, uncomplicated, cheaper cases out of the NHS. Were you to have multiple health problems, you would not have the 'choice' of ISTC care because they deal in the lowest risk cases.[21] This also biases outcome measures, making it even more difficult to draw a fair comparison between the NHS and ISTCs – more complex problems are likely to have more complications than straightforward cases. The creation of ISTCs brought unintended outcomes. The presence of ISTCs impacted on doctors in training, with junior surgeons having fewer hip and knee cases that they were able to perform under supervision.[22] Money was spent on shiny new treatment centres for the least complex patients to have routine treatments. The sickest and most complex patients were given no extra choice and, instead of a fair share of this money and investment, were left with an NHS that had many thousand fewer beds because of the ISTCs.

Another farcical political initiative was the 48-hour target to see a GP. This was set up by the Labour government in 2000: all patients had to be offered a GP appointment within 48 hours. What magical thing happens at 48 hours? What suddenly changes? General practices, told that they must comply but given no new resources, managed to fulfil the target only by no longer allowing patients to book ahead with the doctor of their choice. Dr Iona Heath, now the chair of the Royal College of General Practitioners, said the target: 'prioritised an encounter between any patient and any doctor ahead of one between an individual patient and a preferred doctor'.[23] There was no concomitant increase in the number of appointments for patients; there was simply a redistribution. If you are very unwell, you don't want to wait two days to see a doctor. And if you have a long-term problem, you probably want to plan your next visit well ahead, so that you can sort out transport, or work, or a companion to take you. The 48-hour target suited a certain sort of patient, but did not help either people with chronic diseases or those who were acutely ill.

Doctors should be held to account for their actions. So, too, should politicians, but even if they are voted out, the tangle of their legacy is left to strangle the NHS for years to come. Politics takes precedence over evidence. The Private Finance Initiative (PFI) was a new means whereby the private sector invested in public sector infrastructure, including new hospital builds and clinics. One of the first PFI builds, Norfolk and Norwich University Hospital, was contracted to Octagon, a private sector consortium. The House of Commons public accounts committee reported on this deal in 2006, noting that 'just two years after the new hospital opened, Octagon refinanced the project, dramatically increasing its investors' rate of return to over three times the level Octagon had predicted when bidding for the contract'. Why? 'This is taxpayers' money and the risk of this large liability was incurred essentially so that investors could have fatter returns'. Edward Leigh, chair of the committee, described this debacle as the 'unacceptable face of capitalism'.[24] The National Audit Office noted that this one build netted an £81million windfall for private shareholders.[25] In Scotland alone, it was established that, because of interest payments made to PFI contractors, an estimated £2 billion more was being spent than if the buildings had been built and owned by the NHS directly. This extra spending, concluded Professor Alyson Pollock in the *BMJ*, would be met by cuts to clinical spending.[26] Even the most optimistic politician could not imagine being in power at the end of the 30- or 60-year terms of PFI contracts, meaning that responsibility will never be satisfactorily apportioned.

Or handwashing. In 2007 the *BMJ* said that 'each year in England around 7,000 inpatients have methicillin-resistant *Staphylococcus aureus* (MRSA) bacteraemia and more than 50,000 inpatients aged 65 years and over have *Clostridium difficile* infections.[27] There was frequent media concern that hospitals were dirty places to be. The National Patient Safety Agency, a branch of the Department of Health, launched a 'wash your hands' campaign in 2005.[28] When historians analyse photographs of politicians visiting NHS sites at the turn of the 21st century, they will note that each one, smiling for the cameras, rolls up sleeves and uses copious amounts of alcohol hand gel before entering a ward. Politicians learned to love handwashing. Handwashing became a political dogma that did not involve simply telling people in hospitals to wash their hands often, but also employed nurses to trail staff and audit their handwashing times, hand out badges to 'good' staff and make staff watch DVDs about the proper way to wash their hands. Staff were told to wear badges instructing patients to 'Ask me if my hands are clean', with the aim to 'empower patients, enabling them to take some responsibility for their care'.[29] There was no guidance on what illiterate, blind or unconscious patients were meant to do, but the Hammersmith Hospital hired an entertainer on stilts and 'hand reflexology sessions' to attract attention to its campaign. The Department of Health 'Uniforms and Workwear' policy recommended a 'bare below the elbows' dress code for clinical staff in 2007.[30] Milton Keynes nurses made a 'Clean hands rap' video at a cost of £1,800, urging staff to 'Clean their fingers, just in case the bad bug lingers'.[31]

But was a lack of handwashing and inappropriate clothing amongst hospital staff really the primary problem? The evidence about infections patients acquired in hospitals was always much less about telling staff to roll up their sleeves and much more about a lack of useful investment in hospitals. The evidence the Department of Health cited, correctly, said: 'There is no conclusive evidence that uniforms (or other work clothes) pose a significant hazard in terms of spreading infection.'[30] Hospitals used to employ their own cleaners, with Matron as effective line manager. Over the past decade, cleaning has been franchised out to independent companies, contracted to specific tasks – rather than what Matron insists on. Does this mean worse, or less efficient cleaning as some authors have claimed?[32] A review published in the *American Journal of Infection Control* in 2008 concluded: 'There is a lack of rigorous evidence linking specific hand hygiene interventions with the prevention of HCAIs' (healthcare-associated infections).[33] Indeed, it is the places that aren't, nowadays, regularly cleaned in hospitals where bugs are found: 42% of the curtains around beds are contaminated with bacteria resistant to many types of antibiotic, such as vancomycin-resistant enterococci, and 22% with MRSA, for example.[34] The *Lancet Infectious Diseases* published a paper in 2008 showing that hospital overcrowding and understaffing were culpable for high MRSA rates in Australia;[35] this had been shown in UK hospitals in 2005.[36]

Meanwhile, 'enhanced cleaning' — including not just the standard things but also lockers, all clinical equipment, door handles, chairs, and leaflet racks — being done twice or three times a day produced a decrease in MRSA total aerobic colony counts (contamination rates) of 32.5%. This was done with the addition of one extra cleaner onto a ward.[37] Politically, admitting that competition for cleaning services in the NHS has failed is problematic. It is far easier for politicians to fund a 'fun' PR campaign than to tackle their failure to commission decent cleaning, adequate bed numbers and proper staffing. The people estimated to die every year in England alone partly or solely due to hospital-acquired infection[38] did not do so just because of a lack of handwashing. Blaming hospital infections on a lack of handwashing is to dismiss the evidence.

So, what if the NHS did not take up political ideas unless they were evidence based, properly piloted and proven to produce advantages to patients, including the most vulnerable? What if the NHS were to be charged to find the most cost-effective interventions for patients, and allowed to find the best way of doing them? The NHS is one of the largest organisations in the world, and it is fuelled by people working in it who, free of charge and just because they can, delight in making improvements in what they do, work out better systems to get good results, and who are keen to collaborate and share, not compete. The NHS is an unusual organism, for it does not just evolve to survive but it refills itself regularly with staff who join out of vocation and a desire to serve. Take Renal PatientView, a system that allows patients to view their test results and hospital notes online. This was envisioned and created by doctors and their colleagues with a small amount of external help, and costs a few thousand pounds per renal unit. It allows access to notes and results for patients who wish it, is filled with relevant information, and is popular with both patients and staff.[39] People who work in the NHS for 30 or 40 years want their services to work better because they personally, and the patients in front of them, will benefit.

Evidence-based politics does not yet exist. Politicians are eager to cite evidence when it suits them, of course, but they do not routinely ask for systematic reviews before publishing policy. It is a waste of our common resources to try to provide evidence-based medicine while the vagaries of political will push and pull the service that patients get and the activities that healthcare workers do.

16

The unseen benefits of professional healthcare

The political reach on healthcare goes deep. Politics are capable of insinuating themselves into the subtleties of the interaction between patients and doctors, from how a disclosure of depression is handled to an opinion on where best to get an operation done. This causes a raft of problems; one is that the relationships patients have with their healthcare professionals are full of things 'happening' that might not be easily measurable, or obviously useful.

One of these is the placebo effect. 'Placebo' has come to mean a 'dummy pill', which connotes something derisory about the person who takes it, as though they can be fooled by some kind of 'trick' when they wrongly believe that they have been given something 'real'. When the patient feels better, he has been misled by the belief that the 'medicine' would 'work', when it was, in fact, a 'sham'.

I, and I hope you, immediately dislike this scenario. Doctors should not be magicians or conmen. Neither should the patient feel disbelieved, fobbed off or dismissed with a flick of the pen across the prescription pad.

In day-to-day clinical practice, placebo effects are often useful. They also must be accounted for in clinical studies, or else you will think your 'treatment' is much better than it is. The opposite effect also exists: the 'nocebo' — an inert substance that makes us feel sick.

Take the colour of a pill. We might consider this to be innocuous, insignificant or even boring. But no: green and blue tablets have more sedative effects on patients, and red or orange pills are found to be more stimulatory.[1] This was demonstrated nicely in a group of medical students with a predicted sedative effect with blue tablets or a stimulant effect with pink ones. The pills contained equal amounts of a biologically inert substance, yet more tablets produced more effect.[2]

The placebo effect doesn't just happen with tablets. It also happens with surgical procedures. Arthroscopy is an examination of a joint, most commonly knee, hip or shoulder, using a telescopic instrument. Under anaesthetic, the 'keyhole' instrument can also be used to wash out the joint with saline. When a group of patients with troubling knee symptoms had either 'real' arthroscopy, when the wash-out was performed, or sham surgery, with incisions made in the knee but no wash-out, the effects were the same. Both sets of patients had less pain and better use of their knee after their operations. The 'real' procedure did not give better results.[3] This effect was even tested in heart bypass for angina – an operation that is commonly done and considered very useful, reported back in 1960. The 'real' operation worked – but so did sham surgery. Patients reported a similar reduction in angina after either procedure.[4]

Do some things get better by themselves? Certainly. Voltaire was on the money: 'The art of medicine consists in amusing the patient while nature cures the disease.' Time truly is a marvellous thing in medicine, both for making diagnoses and excluding them. The human body deals well with enormous amounts of insults, be they viral, bacterial, self-inflicted, environmental, or simply bad luck. Sometimes no treatment is the best treatment. Treatments that are unnecessary often mean the doctor looks good, taking credit for improvement when it was simply time that made the difference. This only holds if there are no side-effects of treatment, of course, in which case the doctor will hope that you will view this as a necessary inconvenience in getting better.

It's only through randomised controlled trials that we can learn when it is safe to do nothing and when we should reasonably take action. RCTs mean we can be more sure that our treatment works independent of what was going to happen in any case. But doing absolutely nothing is not going to give you a placebo effect. In our knee arthroscopy trial, above, we would have to compare sham surgery with 'real' surgery (and doesn't that seem a false nomenclature, since they had the same measured effect?) and also with nothing at all, just observing our patient from a distance, with no input and no 'care'.

We can't ignore placebo effects in healthcare. What does this mean in practice? Take, for example, using branded headache tablets (which are usually given flashy packaging and a positive, helpful sounding name) as opposed to generic tablets (in plain packs bearing just their medical denominator). In 1981 the *BMJ* published a study showing that in 835 women with headache, branded 'real' tablets worked better than unbranded 'real' tablets. And branded placebo tablets worked better than unbranded placebo, which worked, overall, worst.[5] The branding and the packaging had a measurable, beneficial effect on headache.

Similarly, better information about interventions may make us feel differently about them. Another trial randomised 48 young adults to an exercise programme, with one group told it was designed to make them feel better about themselves and the other group told this was just an exercise programme. The exercise programmes were identical and so was the two groups' improvement in fitness — but only the individuals who were told that exercise had a beneficial effect on their psychological wellbeing reported this improvement.[6]

The nocebo effect, by contrast, makes us feel worse. A study in Norway examined people who reported headaches when using their mobile phone. The researchers exposed them to phones with active radio frequency signals or none at all. Yet people had their 'mobile phone headache' whether or not the radio signals were active. Their headaches were real; the relationship of their headache to radio frequency producing phones was not.[7]

Well, you may think, we can all expect discomfort in certain situations. The clenching of the jaw and fear as we approach the dentist's waiting room may not help the pain that we experience. We react like Pavlov's dog, so expectant of pain that we feel it, whether or not there is a direct cause.[8]

The *Lancet* published a paper examining the age at death of Chinese-Americans and white Americans. Almost 30,000 Chinese Americans' health records were compared to more than 400,000 'white' controls. In traditional Chinese astrology, a person's year of birth associates that person with a particular health issue. 'Fire people', for example, are susceptible to heart disease, and 'earth people' to tumours. If a Chinese-American had a birth year and a disease considered linked in Chinese astrological belief, then he or she was more likely to die younger. The researchers tried to find other ways to explain this phenomenon but were unable to. 'We conclude that our findings result at least partly from psychosomatic processes,' they wrote.[9] Chinese and Japanese culture associates the number four with death; there is a peak in death rates in Japanese and Chinese people on the fourth day of the month which is not found with white control groups.[10]

'Psychosomatic' has the ring of the fake about it. The term is contemporarily used in a derogatory way, with the implication that people who have such a reaction are somehow psychologically weak, or easily misled. Yet psychosomatic reactions – which I think of as the interplay between a person's psychological and physical state – can have fatal consequences, hardly the result of a weak-willed person or medical trick. People who have depression after a heart attack have been shown to have an increased death rate even when researchers have adjusted their results to take account of factors like social class, smoking or severity of illness.[11] The same link between depression and earlier death was found after heart bypass surgery: depression, even when adjusted for other factors, was an independent risk factor for earlier death. About 19% of patients who were persistently depressed died during follow-up, compared with 10% of patients who were never depressed.[12]

It's fair to say that we don't really know why. Perhaps stress hormones play a role. Take patients with Parkinson's disease, which causes shaking of the limbs. When patients were told that they were likely to receive active medication, their brain scan showed a bigger release of dopamine, even if the medication they were given was a placebo and biologically inactive. When patients were given the same inert placebo and told that it was an inactive drug, there was no similar brain release of dopamine. Dopamine is involved in the 'reward' centres in the brain, and is also central to the treatment of Parkinson's disease.[13] This 'placebo' is useful and relevant. The effect is as real as we can hope for. There is nothing airy-fairy or psychologically weak about it.

There is more. A group of researchers writing in the journal *Pain* examined patients after major chest surgery. They were given a continuous saline drip, plus other painkillers, which they could freely have on request. Plain saline has no effect on pain. There were three study groups. The first group was not told about the effect of the drip. The second group was given the same saline but told that it may or may not be a powerful analgesic. The third group was told that the saline was actually a powerful painkiller. The second group reduced their use of painkillers overall compared with the first group, but the third group had the lowest use of all.[14] What we think is happening affects what actually does happen.

We get a clue from another study, this time examining the effect of naloxone on placebo pain relief. Naloxone is a drug used to reverse the effects of opiate drugs, which can be so strong that the overdosed person can stop breathing. It's commonly used in A&E if a drug user is comatose after an overdose of heroin.

In this study, again from the journal *Pain*, people were deliberately given painful arms. They were then treated with an injection of saline, which has no effect on pain, but the participants were told it was pain relief. This injection was a placebo pain reliever. Next a dose of naloxone was injected. This resulted in people complaining of more pain. The researchers concluded that 'endogenous opioids' – the opiates we produce ourselves within our brains – 'are involved in producing a placebo-induced analgesia.'[15] Placebo effects can be real and chemical – as chemical and real as anything else we do.

This stuff is not just fascinating. It's relevant to the nuts and bolts of what happens in medicine. Whether you want to call these phenomena psychological effects, or behavioural effects, or placebo effects, they exist, and they have to be accounted for whenever medicine is practised.

Placebo effect without placebo?

There is another problem with placebos. It may be that the case for a placebo 'working' is, or has been, overstated. Cochrane researchers think that because placebo is not often compared properly to both doing nothing at all (not even a placebo) and active treatment, it is difficult to disentangle the placebo effect from simple waiting – a general improvement over time.[16]

Waiting for improvements is often difficult for doctors and patients. Often, time is all that is needed for straightforward and uncomplicated health problems to go away. Some headaches, most colds, most flu, most gastroenteritis, most inflamed insect bites and most cuts and bruises don't need specific treatment. Some stress, anxiety, and low mood will also settle by itself. Your body, designed to deal with numerous insults, will often sort you out with no recourse to anything except time.

Of course, when a doctor prescribes something or a patient takes a remedy, it is tempting to ascribe any benefits to the treatment and not the natural course of events. This makes doctors feel that they are doing the right thing and the next time a similar illness unfolds, they will feel justified in repeating their actions – after all, it worked the last time!

Placebo effects are not the same thing as a placebo pill or sham operation. A placebo is inert, but the placebo effect is not.

A detailed review about placebo effects in the *Lancet* in 2010 suggested: 'Evidence indicates that the placebo effect is a genuine psychobiological phenomenon attributable to the overall therapeutic context. The psychosocial context surrounding the patient can be comprised of both individual patient and clinician factors, and the interaction between the patient, clinician, and treatment environment. The latter represents the many factors involved in a treatment context (such as the specific nature of the treatment and the way it is administered) and the 'Doctor-Patient Relationship' which is a term that encompasses a host of factors that constitute the therapeutic interaction.'[17]

Philosophers and psychologists have written volumes on what the placebo effect 'means' and whether or not it can be used ethically, without lying to patients. There seems a massive vexation as to whether healthcare professionals, working in normal day to day practice, can or should ever lie about whether or not patients are given placebo tablets, for example.

The professional discomfort about placebo medication can be traced back a century, when medical journals were arguing about when deception was and wasn't appropriate. Placebos had been described as a 'pious fraud' and could be coloured water, bread pills, or ash; Richard Cabot, professor at Harvard Medical School, said at the beginning of the 20th century that he used to give placebos 'by the bushels'.[18] Doctors didn't have many useful treatments to offer anyone at that time (and it could be argued that placebos were less harmful than some of the treatments that could be offered). In 1954 an anonymous article in the *Lancet* stated: 'For some unintelligent or inadequate patients life is made easier by a bottle of medicine to comfort their ego; that to refuse a placebo to a dying incurable patient may be simply cruel; and that to decline the humour of an elderly 'chronic' brought up on the bottle is hardly within the bounds of possibility.'[19]

Let's put placebos, the sugar pill, and the pretend operation to one side. Let's concentrate on placebo effects, which are, by definition, good. Patronisingly deceiving people is not. Can the modern patient and the professional doctor have one without the other?

I think so. Good doctors can generate placebo effects – but they don't need to use placebos.

Concomitant professional outcomes

We have already seen that if patients are given good information about possible positive effects, for example in the exercise and self-esteem trial, they are more likely to report that benefit. We know that giving branded painkillers can have a beneficial effect on pain relief. These would be simple enough to use in everyday general practice. Placebo effects can add value to healthcare but in these examples, there is no 'sham', and no lying or deception.

Thinking and reading about these 'other effects' that happen when patients interact with healthcare facilities, I first wondered if the placebo effect should instead be called 'caring effects' because there is much to do with the effects of a 'caring' doctor-patient relationship within them. But I'm worried that 'caring effects' sounds wishy-washy and benign, unlike the powerful and useful real effects they are capable of. I'm instead going to settle for the mouthful of 'concomitant professional outcomes'. This matters because professional healthcare should be able to use the 'clean power' that these effects bring. But the political push towards managing medics by tickbox and protocol excoriates the latent power of the consultation.

Bear with me.

Take people with irritable bowel syndrome. This condition causes disrupted bowel habit, often with cramping pains and urgency: it is chronic, and common. A trial examined the effect of treating 262 people with the condition, dividing them into three groups. One group remained on the waiting list and was simply monitored. The other two groups received sham acupuncture – that is, use of needles that did not concur with any of the theories or taught acupuncture courses. One group had acupuncture performed in a 'limited interaction' with the therapist. The other received, as part of the sham acupuncture, a warm, empathetic practitioner, who sought a positive relationship with the patient.[21]

The results: 28% of patients on the waiting list reported adequate relief from their symptoms – time got them better. Irritable bowel syndrome tends to relapse and recur, so this isn't surprising. Of the basic acupuncture group, 44% of the patients had adequate control of their symptoms – which seems impressive until you find that 62% of the patients who had the warm, empathetic practitioner got adequate pain relief.[20]

We could argue that it is unethical to withhold humane and supportive communication from patients for all kinds of reasons. This is evidence that a good relationship with a healthcare professional can make people feel better. No matter how many computer systems we want to crowd into a doctor's office, no matter how many guidelines and clever diagnosing and complex statistics we want to cite, in real life things are different. We are human together, and that relationship can bring dividends.

Back in 1987, one doctor studied a group of patients who had undefined and undiagnosed symptoms. Such a scenario is common in general practice. These patients had no abnormalities on physical examination nor laboratory tests. They were divided into four groups. Two groups had 'positive' consultations, where the patient was given a diagnosis and told he or she was likely to get better quickly. The other two groups had 'negative' consultations, where no diagnosis or prognosis was given. One of the 'positive' groups had a prescription given, as did one of the 'negative' groups. The 'treatment' given was the vitamin thiamine, intended to act as a placebo. The difference was marked. Of patients who had a 'positive' consultation, 64% described themselves as being better in two weeks compared to 39% who had a 'negative' consultation. There was no difference with the placebo pills. It appeared that the tone of the consultation made a difference to how patients felt and how their symptoms progressed.[21]

That particular study was done out of concern that doctors who shared uncertainty with their patients might dull the effect of 'doctor as drug', where the doctor is seen as the 'healer'. I'd rather see it as 'caring effects' or, better, concomitant professional outcomes, where a skilled doctor is aware of the potential effects of the consultation and harnesses them for ethical benefit.

Other studies have tried to demonstrate that specific qualities in consultations have a beneficial effect on patients. One trend is to measure the degree of 'patient-centredness' in a consultation. This is said to include things like discussing the illness and the patient's concerns and expectations – dealing with the whole person and not just the disease, and 'enhancing the doctor-patient relationship'. These phrases teeter too far towards jargon for my taste, but we should not ignore the message. A study published in the *BMJ* showed that if the doctor was interested in the patient, positive, and clear in communication, patients were more satisfied with the consultation, as well as more enabled to deal with their illness. If doctors failed in the consultation, patients were likely to suffer symptoms for longer and to have unnecessary referrals made to hospital.[22]

To a certain extent this should be common sense. If you are unwell and bewildered, confused, badly informed, and don't know how to deal with symptoms or illness, it hardly bodes well. It's easy to imagine more need for urgent or emergency care, more anxiety and more pain or discomfort than need be. The point should not be missed: the individual patient should be at the centre of what we are doing.

That should seem obvious, surely? Sadly, it is not. When a patient arrives and I put her name into the computer, her 'missed' smears and unmeasured blood pressures pop up on the screen. There are stop smoking quotas to be hit and flu vaccinations to do. The orientation of general practice has become attuned to the march of the GP contract and government priorities. The patient's voice, waiting to describe symptoms, the impact on her work, or the worries that they could mean something sinister, can be easily muffled as doctors think they are doing good work by concentrating on targets instead. But these targets are government work, not patients' priorities.

What would happen if doctors started to ignore government priorities and concentrated on the concerns of the patient with them? Two similar practices were compared, however, one had longer consultations than the other. The practice with longer appointment times reaped dividends. Patients returned less often and fewer prescriptions were dispensed.[23] Another study has shown that longer consultation times were related to better quality of care.[24] A systematic review in the *British Journal of General Practice* in 2002 concluded: 'Patients seeking help from a doctor who spends more time with them are more likely to have a consultation that includes important elements of care.'[25] Yet, as socio-economic deprivation worsens, so too does psychological distress – but consultation length with GPs working in these areas is shorter.[26] But when extra time was given to patients visiting their GPs, the patients became more able and understanding of what was happening to them. Doctors became less stressed and more able to plan better for their patients' conditions.[27]

We can dismiss deceptive sugar pills and use other, more ethical and equitable means of putting human values into healthcare. Professionalism must reject paternalistic placebos; but professionals must care about patients.

The meaning of holism

I have not attempted to discuss alternative or complementary medicine in this book: I find the division into orthodox and complementary unhelpful. Medical interventions are either evidence based or not. If a medicine works, it is not complementary – it is just medicine. Some medicines, like routine steroids for head injury as previously described, may have been prescribed by mainstream doctors but they didn't work and did do harm. St John's Wort, meanwhile, is a 'herbal' medicine that is chemically similar to the SSRI antidepressant fluoxetine and has been shown to be more effective than placebo in mild to moderate depression.[28] Effectiveness, safety and acceptability should have the same standards regardless of the provenance of the therapy.

Many people in the developed world, and who have a choice about treatments for illnesses, choose from the selection of non-evidence-based treatments, such as homoeopathy or herbal medicine. Surveys suggest that between 3.1% and 24.9% of patients in the UK who have cancer use herbal preparations.[29] One survey in the US found that 40% of people had used a complementary therapy in the previous year; no wonder that an estimated 425 million visits to alternative therapists occur annually.[30] Why? The survey found that people visiting alternative therapists were not particularly unhappy with conventional medicine. However agreeing with the statement 'the health of my body, mind and spirit are related, and whoever cares for my health should take that into account' was highly predictive of using alternative medicine. Higher educational achievement, not lower, predicted more use of non-evidence-based treatments. 'A subset of individuals may be attracted to these nontraditional therapies because they find in them an acknowledgement of the importance of treating illness within a larger context of spirituality and life meaning.'

I don't think doctors should attempt to be priests, or chaplains. Yet the understanding of what illness and disability mean to a person is fundamental to supporting and tailoring medical care to that person. This is what truly 'person centred' care should be about. It would be dreadful if the only way the unwell person was to receive this understanding was in the alternative sector, far away from evidence, and as a fee-paying customer, not a patient.

How can doctors ethically offer this deeper kind of dimension to patients? Part of good medical professional behaviour is trying to offer continuity. This means that a patient and doctor have knowledge of each other from past consultations and expect to have ongoing contact. From a patient's point of view, this can mean that they do not have to 'start at the beginning' of their story at every visit. It means that the doctor already has an appreciation of that person's priorities and work or social background.

When people have minor, 'low impact' symptoms they are more likely to prefer quick access with any GP. But when patients have long-standing conditions, or difficulty dealing with an uncertain problem, they prefer to wait to see their usual doctor.[31] It's easy to see, yet again, how people who are more sick become most disadvantaged; they would be least likely to benefit from the numerous providers offering 'minor illness' services. Again, a study in the *British Journal of General Practice* in 2001 concluded, from a series of questionnaires and/or interviews with almost 1,000 patients and 300 GPs, that a personal doctor-patient relationship was highly valued by patients and doctors, especially for more serious family issues and psychological problems.[32]

Continuity of care is not just preferred by patients and doctors:

it can also reduce health spending. In the US state of Delaware, more continuity of care was associated with fewer hospital admissions.[33] Seeing the same doctor for long-term conditions like asthma[34] or diabetes[35] reduces the need for urgent or inpatient care.[36] For patients at the end of life with terminal cancer, greater family doctor continuity of care was associated with less need for urgent out-of-hours care.[39] It isn't just hospital admissions or emergency calls that are reduced. A longitudinal study in the US, observing almost 13,000 patients who had 1,000 hospital admissions and 240,000 prescriptions, found that continuity of care reduced all costs: for each additional doctor or nurse involved, more money was added in terms of prescription costs and outpatient visits.[37] Continuity of care is a straightforward, ethical way of improving health.

So continuity of care benefits patients and taxpayers. Despite this, a high level of continuity of care is routinely denied to – as usual – the most unwell patients. This has been caused and exacerbated by politics.

Here is a rheumatologist, writing to the *BMJ* in 2011 with his experience of working with PFI hospitals in his area in London.

'My hospital can no longer deal with medical emergencies, and the withdrawal of all intensive care means that complex or high risk surgery cannot be done. I can no longer admit emergencies from outpatients, but have to ask colleagues at other sites to take them over. The use of medical beds as a 'step-down' facility has led to early and inappropriate transfers from acute sites and has been bad for continuity of care and length of stay.'[38]

The organisational structure created through political ideology neither recognised nor encouraged his continuing responsibility for his patients, who, when they became more unwell, were simply transferred elsewhere. The slogan 'no decision about me without me' is thus demonstrated as worthless. The sickest patients are not offered meaningful 'choice' about where they will be treated. The very nature of general practice has been altered by politicians who think that convenience must trump all else. While no patient should be forced to see a particular doctor, the dissolution of GPs' personal lists of patients in favour of a 'practice list' has meant each GP is less likely to be responsible for named patients. So, too, have the Coalition's plans to enable anyone to register with any GP no matter where they live. This is likely to increase meaningful choice only for people with minor illness, who we already know are flexible about who they see for diagnosis and treatment. But for people with more complex or enduring problems, there is no evidence that they want – or will benefit from – this option.

Holistic care should mean continuity. In mental health, patients are encouraged to write 'advance care plans' that can be used in case of illness. Yet the doctors responsible for patients with mental illness are often not allowed to take responsibility for them through crises. For a person who is mentally unwell, it can be difficult to fairly discuss treatment interventions. In cases of mental illness, a knowledge of the person when well can be very helpful. It is easier for the doctor to recognise a change in the person's mental state, and to know what his preferences for treatments are. If, for example, the patient has made it plain at consultations over the past year that he would, or would not, want electroconvulsive therapy, this can be factored into his care. Similarly, continuity of care makes it more likely that GPs will diagnose depression accurately.[39] And patients themselves value 'the importance of building a continuing relationship with one person over time. Frequent changes in healthcare providers and repeatedly reviewing medical histories were frustrating.'[40]

Yet the size and structure of the modern mental health team can make continuity an impossibility. The team may include 'psychiatrists, community psychiatric nurses, social workers, occupational therapists, clinical psychologists, pharmacists, team managers, approved mental health professionals, receptionists, secretaries, outreach workers, benefits workers, support workers, recovery workers, vocational therapists, art therapists and psychotherapists.'[41] A group of psychiatrists, writing in the *British Journal of Psychiatry*, wrote about how it was:

'. . . easy to understand how we have arrived at the model of distributed responsibility and leadership as a pragmatic, short term response to recent crises in staffing and morale in general psychiatry. However, we should not assume that this pragmatic emergency 'solution' is an ideal, or even desirable state of affairs. Although distributed responsibility may make life easier for psychiatrists and appears to be the cheaper option, it does not follow that this is in the best interests of patients. Should we now be arguing for better evidence-based services and the resources and workforce to deliver these services? We suggest a useful thought experiment: if a member of your family were a patient, is a distributed responsibility the one for which you would opt?'[42]

The ludicrous paradox of being a modern patient is underlined yet again: the more ill you are, the less help you get. People with significant mental illness, and who are in need of diagnosis and treatment, are referred to as – and this is supposedly empowering – 'service users', even when most would prefer to be called patients.[43] Psychiatric care is most effective and better for patients when it is kept to a small team, but the 2011 White Paper proposes that individual parts of the 'patient journey' be franchised out, via GP commissioning, to the most competitive bidder. This is despite academic evidence that more competition between hospitals, as seen in the 1990s under the Conservatives, reduces quality of care and increases mortality rates.[44]

In fact, we already know that this kind of fragmentation – one service for a psychologist, another for prescriptions, another for social support – is bad for patients. Citing the previous tendering out of addiction services to 'any willing provider', one spokesman for the Royal College of Psychiatrists described 'a pathway of care that is very fragmented, with one provider for detoxification services, one for social support etc. Writ large across the NHS, that would lead to a real deterioration in care. Would you want one provider for community psychiatric nurses? Would you want another for psychological input?' A social worker was clear: 'I can see it all becoming more chaotic.'[45] Indeed, the Royal College of Psychiatrists expressed its opinion on the Coalition proposals:

'We are particularly concerned to avoid fragmentation of services with several providers delivering different aspects of a care pathway – these providers constantly changing as services are re-tendered. The re-tendering of services from one provider to another risks poor continuity of care for those recipients of care who have long term conditions and who would therefore be subject to numerous transfers of care as the treatment provider changes hands. Competition alone without quality can lead to a system which is highly complex and difficult for providers and service users to understand. There have been many occasions where the frequent re-tendering of services has been highly disruptive for patients . . . patients are falling through gaps during the re-tendering process and there have been reports of untoward clinical incidents as a result of poor continuity of care . . .'[46]

Competitive tendering will mean, in practice, for a cancer patient, that his chemotherapy will be administered at a site far away from his regular oncology nurse, who in turn works for a different provider from his oncologist, who is again in a different service from his radiotherapist. The plans for 'any willing provider' to tender to supply NHS services means that the more complex our care, the less likely it is that all of our health professionals will be working from the same base unit. Should it really become the responsibility of sick patients to manage their own care and make sure they see the right people at the right time? Is this kind of administrative co-ordination really the kind of 'choice' that patients should be grateful for?

We are missing an enormous opportunity to do better for patients, using basic professional skills and simple humanity. If continuity of care came in a capsule and was sold as a drug, one can only imagine the enormous lengths to which the pharmaceutical company responsible would go to tell doctors, politicians and patients about this useful, low-cost and safe intervention. But because politicians tend to place political ideology before evidence, and because the evidence says that continuing care is a concomitant professional outcome, and not something easily tendered, bought or sold, it fails to get much publicity or be taken seriously.

17

Getting back to the right kind of care

While doctors should, therefore, be concentrating their efforts on doing their best for patients who are sick, they are encouraged by Department of Health lucre to screen and diagnose people with illnesses who are not unwell and have no symptoms of illness.

When we consider the raw deal that people who are actually sick get, the growing emphasis on finding and treating people who are not unwell creates two major problems. First, treating more well patients diverts resources from unwell patients. Second, when we diagnose and treat asymptomatic conditions or risk factors, we necessarily treat far more people than will benefit.

Numbers like high blood pressure or cholesterol levels don't have a clear distinction between 'normal' or not. The push towards catching well people in the disease net has resulted in labels designed to capture more people. So, if a blood pressure or glucose level is normal, the person could still have 'pre-hypertension' or 'pre-diabetes' – even when their numbers are ones that are considered normal.

Yet 'lifestyle modification' is simply attention to diet, exercise and weight: exactly what would be said to any person without 'pre-hypertension' seeking advice about their health. What is the evidence that making a diagnosis of 'pre-hypertension' will benefit patients? One pharmacologist, reviewing the evidence, wrote: 'The vast majority have low absolute risk and whether drug treatment would be beneficial is uncertain. . . any change in recommendations should await adequately powered outcome studies.'[2] Not everyone has been so keen to insist on evidence that diagnosing more 'pre-illness' serves us well. The chief executive of Diabetes UK has said that pre-diabetes is a 'ticking time-bomb . . . it's staggering that seven million people in the UK have pre-diabetes, which is often a precursor to type 2 diabetes . . .'[3] Estimates in the US predict that half of US citizens will have type 2 diabetes or 'pre-diabetes' by 2020;[4] however, it is clear that, as the US Preventive Services Taskforce wrote in 2008, 'direct evidence is lacking on the health benefits of detecting type 2 diabetes by either targeted or mass screening'.[5] Treating pre-diabetes is best done by attention to the usual evidence-based lifestyle criteria (weight, stopping smoking, diet and exercise.) While some work suggests that treatment with metformin, a tablet used to treat diabetes, might slow the progression of pre-diabetes into diabetes in some people, it is not certain that it actually prevents the disease.[6] The best advice for a healthy lifestyle remains uncomplicated.

In Scotland, where heart disease is especially common,[7] attempts have been made to compensate and use risk calculations loaded against living in high-risk areas. This means, that even if you are a football-playing, slim, healthy-eating and non-smoking male, if you add a postcode for a 'high risk' area – much of Glasgow – the risk is calculated as higher which means it is more likely that drugs such as statins will be prescribed than if a postcode was entered for a lower risk environment.

This is troubling. What causes early deaths in some areas of the country as opposed to others? Why do some populations seem to die sooner than others?

Michael Marmot is a public health doctor who has sought to find out. In the *Lancet*, in 2005, he examined international factors causing early deaths throughout the world. He listed: social gradient, stress, poor circumstances in early life, social exclusion, work, unemployment, social support, addiction, food and transport as social determinants of health.

'But would it be helpful to go into a deprived Australian Aboriginal population and point out that they should really take better care of themselves – that their smoking and obesity were killing them; and if they must drink, please do so in moderation? Unlikely. To borrow Geoffrey Rose's term, we need to examine the causes of the causes . . . although it might be obvious that poverty is at the root of much of the problem of infectious disease, and needs to be solved, it is less obvious to break the link between poverty and disease.'[8]

Treating poverty with pills

How should breaking down the divisions between poverty and disease be done? Is giving out pills to treat cholesterol, possibly reducing one risk factor for cardiovascular disease slightly, really the best way to reduce inequalities in health? When we use funds in one place, we cannot use them in another. Is it useful to treat poverty with pills?

Perhaps not. Instead, medicalising poverty may reinforce the patient paradox. The National Cholesterol Education Program in the US found that 'many of those who participate in public screening programmes have been previously tested, fall into low-benefit groups, or fail to comply with recommended follow-up'.[9] People who have been told they are at high cardiovascular risk are more likely to recall their risk levels to be lower.[10] There is, again, a paradox: people who are least likely to benefit from cholesterol screening will seek screening and take treatment. People at higher risk of early death are less likely to be screened or treated for high cholesterol. As a method of trying to deal with the highest risk people first, cholesterol screening fails.

Focusing just on cholesterol means that it is easy to disregard other important contributors to ill health. A report from the Community Health Exchange in Scotland said, in 2004:

'Although it has been proven that many low-income families do try to improve the diet of their children by buying wholemeal bread, fresh fruit, vegetables and pasta, the high cost of trying to feed your family day to day makes it impossible not to buy the more filling high fat and sugar-laden foods. To wander around a glossy supermarket with very little money in your purse, it's a little wonder that this leads to depression, a sense of never coping and always having to make a choice between heating your home or buying a wholesome varied diet for your family. It's a constant battle, leading to low self-esteem and a feeling of helplessness and despair.'[11]

Is it right to treat the outcomes of poverty with medicine, when the real sources of preventable diseases are social and political? Some people may think that there is little point in using drugs to delay their death from cardiac disease just to endure a longer quantity of poor quality of life. When doctors are considering their role in society, this has to be addressed. Are doctors guilty of colluding in the belief that prescriptions can treat poverty? Isn't this an obscene sticking plaster?

Pharmaceutical products cannot be the answer to social exclusion. Using tablets to try to reverse social damage makes patients, rather than valued citizens, out of people. Medicalising poverty is a simplistic and superficial way of dealing with larger problems. So the insistent GP contract boxes flash up on the computer screen, insisting on cholesterols and blood pressures being measured even when the patient is disclosing other, entirely different fears about the here and now. The doctor can become distracted. The patient's problem can become lost.

Single issue subversions

Every day there is a new health matter we are told we're not 'aware' enough about – breast, bowel and prostate cancer award themselves whole awareness months. Most just get a day – the Sexual Dysfunction Association has a 'Think about Sex' day on February 14th. Eating disorders, salt, ovarian cancer, glaucoma, kidneys, endometriosis, dystonia, ME, lupus, cystic fibrosis and hypertension, hepatitis, sexual health, stroke, even antibotics and tinnitus, all boast awareness days of their own, when press releases are sent, case studies are offered to journalists, and experts are available to take over the airwaves and newspapers.

All healthcare charities wish for more attention than they currently get from citizens, politicians, journalists and healthcare professionals. Some, as we have seen, have funding from pharmaceutical companies. We have become so inured to the 'need' for awareness that most people never bother questioning whether it is a good idea to receive information about our health this way. Most people who hear the call to awareness will never have the disease or disorder in question, and the evidence-based messages about what can improve your quality and quantity of life – not smoking, drinking moderately, being a sensible weight and eating well – are drowned out in the clamour. Presumably this is because sensible lifestyle advice will prevent many illnesses, not just one, and presumably because this advice has not changed much over the past half century, it is deemed unnewsworthy.

It's possible, and harmful, to look at medical problems from the wrong end of the telescope. NICE released guidelines in April 2011 on the diagnosis and treatment of ovarian cancer.[12] Ovarian cancer is often difficult to diagnose because the symptoms can be vague – bloating, or pain – and are experienced by many women who do not have the disease. Accurate diagnosis is further hindered because the tests – namely, ultrasound scan and a blood marker for ovarian tumour, Ca-125 – can suggest a problem even when the woman does not have ovarian cancer. Screening programmes designed to detect ovarian cancer in women with no symptoms but at high risk of developing it have not been useful. 'Despite enormous effort,' wrote a US group, 'there is no proof that routine screening for ovarian cancer in either the high-risk or general populations with serum markers, sonograms or pelvic examination decreases mortality.'[13]

The NICE guidelines instigated a change in management for women who attended their doctor with symptoms that could be ovarian cancer, or one of many other diagnoses. Previously, if a woman complained of vague lower abdominal symptoms, an ultrasound scan would be used to assess not just the ovaries, but the uterus, bladder, kidneys, lymph nodes, liver and gallbladder.

NICE decided that doctors should do a Ca-125 blood test first, and only order an ultrasound if the result was high.

However, this guidance is biased towards diagnosis of ovarian cancer and not other serious causes of the same symptoms. NICE itself noted that 0.23% of women with these symptoms of bloating and pain would turn out to have ovarian cancer, meaning that 99.77% would not. So for about 420 women with these symptoms, one would have ovarian cancer.

Finding that woman is not straightforward. Ca-125, a tumour marker, was originally developed and used to monitor the success of therapy for treatment of ovarian cancer and to check for relapse after treatment. If we take a group of 100,000 symptomatic women, and assume that 0.23% of them will have ovarian cancer, that will give us 230 women with ovarian cancer to find. If we do a Ca-125 test on all of them, it will be positive 22,128 times. Almost a fifth of women will have a positive blood test. However, only a tiny proportion will actually have ovarian cancer – only 179 women out of those 22,128. In other words, thousands of women are told they have an abnormal result but only a very few – 0.81% – will actually have ovarian cancer. Nor is the sensitivity of the test very good. A negative Ca-125 result will be returned for 77,821 women. However, 51 of these will have ovarian cancer that won't be picked up through the test. That represents almost a fifth of all women with ovarian cancer.

If ultrasound were to be used as the first test, it would diagnose 196 of the 230 women, with fewer false positives – 16,961, as opposed to 21,949. This NICE guidance – picking off one cause of symptoms rather than holistically reckoning with all of them – is so focused on ovarian cancer that it has demoted all the other potential causes of lower abdominal symptoms in women. Nor is there guidance on what to do when a raised Ca-125 is followed by a normal ultrasound: the evidence gap is cavernous.

What a mess for patients and doctors to sort out! The Guideline Development Group working for NICE contained three representatives from patient groups on the committee that wrote the guidelines, one GP and no public health doctor or epidemiologist. Are these guidelines doing women a favour by swinging away from a broad diagnostic construct to a system focusing exclusively on ovarian cancer? Or have they become skewed by a minority: the fear of ovarian cancer usurping fear of uterine or bowel cancer, kidney stones or bladder abnormalities? Why was the cheaper blood test being used instead of the more expensive ultrasound, even if this generated more false positives? The bottom line is that 99.77% of women who have potentially serious symptoms do not have ovarian cancer – but may have another, possibly just as serious, condition. We surely do not want fear and fervour about ovarian cancer alone to skew medical priorities. We are not even sure about the natural history of ovarian cancer and the Ca-125, as a cancer-screening marker, has been deemed 'best of a bad lot'.[14] We have to make sure we ask the right questions, free from bias and fear of one disease, or else we will never get useful answers about how to improve outcomes from this, or other, diseases.

The truth is that no matter how laudable the aims of a pressure group might be, by definition, it seeks to deflect attention from somewhere else and onto its own cause. It is not possible for attention or awareness to increase continuously. There is a limited number of hours in the day or week. I wonder how 'aware' ovarian cancer groups are of bowel cancer or renal cancer? The push and pull for our attention means that our finite scope for awareness is being drained by pressure groups, while less fashionable but equally important diseases are sidelined.

Test result	Ovarian cancer	Not ovarian cancer	Percentage
Ca-125 positive	179	21,949	0.81%
Ca-125 is negative	51	77,821	0.07%
Ultrasound suspicious	196	16,961	1.14%
Ultrasound normal	34	82,809	0.04%

Ovarian cancer; positives and negatives.

The war on cancer, the battle with disease and death

The pull towards awareness has brought an openness in discussing illness and its sequelae. People live their illnesses online, in newspaper columns or tweets. It's become impossible to read about people who have had a diagnosis of cancer without descriptions of them in a 'battle' or 'war'. Military analogies flourish alongside the 'Big C'. People talk about themselves as 'survivors'; memorial notices say that he or she 'lost a fight' against disease. Giving up is seen as weak, beating illness is strong. Treatments are called 'magic bullets' and therapies deemed 'resistance'.

Partly, this analogy is political in origin, dating to US President Nixon laying down the National Cancer Act in 1971, nicknamed, the 'war on cancer'.[15] It is an analogy with numerous faults that exemplifies the problems of sexed-up medicine.

As we have seen, cancer is a broad description. There are cancers that will co-exist, rather than kill. There are cancers that are amenable to cure, though the treatment may be unpleasant or difficult. And then there are cancers, along with heart conditions, lung disease or neurological disorders, that are malignant in nature and course. Some can be alleviated, others palliated. Sometimes death can be delayed (and we may as well remember that death is *only ever* delayed) and sometimes it is only our symptoms that can be ameliorated. Making 'war' on cancer might not be the most helpful or kind response. In the US, a study was done comparing patients who had lung cancer that had spread. They were divided into two groups. One group was treated with standard chemotherapy, the other group was given the same treatment but with early palliative care. The group receiving palliative care had less aggressive chemotherapy, a better quality of life – and a longer survival time. If palliative care had been a drug, it would be nicknamed a blockbuster. Aggressively seeking a cure in these patients didn't add time to life.[16] There may be disadvantages to staying in hospital too: more treatments, more financial cost, more side-effects, more medicalisation, but no gain.

On the illness battlefield, 'giving up' is a pejorative action.

Should doctors always recommend treatments for their patients no matter how slender the value of the treatment might be, and no matter how difficult to bear the side-effects? Should doctors arm themselves for 'war', never giving up and not allowing disease to 'win'?

There are fault lines here, rendering an illusion of control over our bodies and disease. Every day, people who have lived non-smoking, exercising, healthy-eating lives get nasty diseases through no fault of their own. Every day, despite having endured tedious, nauseating, painful or disfiguring treatment, people still relapse or die from disease. A 'war' implies that diseases can be overcome by effort and will, but the truth about many treatments and many 'cures' is that they do not work terribly well.

The late Christopher Hitchens wrote in *Vanity Fair* magazine in 2011:

'Myself, I love the imagery of struggle. I sometimes wish I was suffering in a good cause, or risking my life for the good of others, instead of just being a gravely endangered patient. Allow me to inform you, though, that when you sit in a room with other finalists, and kindly people bring a huge transparent bag of poison and plug it into your arm, and you either read or don't read a book while the venom sack gradually empties itself into your system, the image of the ardent soldier or revolutionary is the very last one that will occur to you. You feel swamped with passivity and impotence: dissolving in powerlessness like a sugar lump in water.'[17]

A paper consisting of interviews with healthcare staff in the US journal *The Oncologist* noted one nurse: 'I often hear, "If I don't fight hard enough, I am letting my family down."' An oncologist said: 'I think there is a tyranny of positive thinking that goes along with these metaphors. Sometimes, you see it in couples, too, where one person wants to voice their fears and another wants to shut them down. If you don't think positively, bad things are going to happen.' Another doctor, recognising the futility of some 'cancer wars' thought instead:

'There is a rise in narcissism in our culture, and it is often accompanied by fantasy, with the hope that desire will trump reality. We want to live in a microwave culture, where I get what I want instantly and magically, with no struggle and no fight. I don't know about you, but that does not conform to my view of the world. I want my kids to be fighters: I want my patients to be fighters. But, I want them to fight for the right thing. You can fight for courage, loyalty, and living well. I want that little 2-pound kid to be a fighter. I don't have as big a problem with saying 'let's fight'. The question is at what point you are holding on to your metaphor in the wrong fight.'[18]

Is it fair on the most ill people to make them feel that they must take up their weapons for war? I recall, when I was a junior doctor, a ward round with a new consultant who was eager to employ the latest in informed consent. There had been recent media accusations of ageism, with outrage that elderly people were routinely denied cardiopulmonary resuscitation in the event of a cardiac arrest. These people apparently had 'DNR' (do not resuscitate) orders written in their notes. Contemporary medical ethicists had been furious, demanding that old people had as much right to treatment for cardiac arrest as anyone else.

In fact, I see this as a further example of the patient paradox. The more ill you are, the less of the right kind of care you get. On that ward round we visited a frail man. He had been admitted with pneumonia, and had an extensive and serious medical history: a previous stroke, two heart attacks and heart failure. His treatment worked, but slowly and steadily. He gradually regained confidence enough to make a few steps around the bed. After a discussion and an examination, the new consultant asked the man if he wished to be resuscitated should he have a cardiac arrest. The man looked, puzzled, at the doctor. Then a new expression creased his face: he was devastated. His confidence and his hope for getting home evaporated. Explaining the rationale for the guidelines and the need to ask for his views made no difference. His wife, too, was distraught. She had assumed that the doctors and nurses would have always done their best for him, regardless. The following day I discussed the situation with another consultant. Knowing the gentleman's history of heart attacks, heart failure, and stroke, he calculated his likely survival from CPR using several different methods of calculating his risk scores. All of which returned a result of zero chance of survival from resuscitation.

This isn't an argument against helping people make good decisions about their health – just the opposite. The choice being offered to that man was futile. It was no choice at all. If the doctors were to perform resuscitation it would not have helped him. His fragile body would endure cracked ribs and a bruised airway as tubes would be put down his throat. It might benefit doctors, who, in doing 'everything possible', might feel they were beyond criticism. It would have been both more honest, and kinder to ensure that man knew he would be cared for and comforted until his death with no unnecessary pain or discomfort.

And the manner of death? What about the kind of death on offer? Is it always right to have one last round of chemotherapy, spending the week in a hospital bed, rigged up to tubes and swallowing anti-nausea medication? Would it be giving up the 'fight' to decide that there has now been enough treatment, and to come home, to treat symptoms and to comfort? There is such pressure put on patients and their families that they should explore all options, get second, third, or fourth opinions, read up everything online and battle for the very best of care, that we are in danger of forgetting what all the care is for anyway. In fact, a review of the evidence suggested that having a 'fighting spirit' rather than feeling helpless or hopeless does not influence either survival or recurrence of cancer.[19] Isn't this a good thing for people with cancer to know about? Instead, a respondent to this research, rather than feeling liberated from the shackles of battle, wrote: 'Stating definitively that the efforts of the patient can have no such effect has been a source of much unnecessary discouragement to a great many people with cancer.'[20] The truth is, we are trying to control the wrong things.

For many others it is a great relief no longer to deal in the charades and costumes of vigorous positivism. It may be absolutely reasonable to admit fears, draw lines about acceptability of treatment, and live life on our own terms, not those of medical protocol. Lionel Shriver's book *So Much for That* narrates a woman's death from cancer. Finally free from the shackles of chemotherapy, she dies surrounded by her family, at home, at peace and even with joy at a life well lived. For those of us who have witnessed the desperation for 'a cure', the complications of interventions, and the nausea, discomfort and bruising nature of them, calling time on futile 'cures' is hard. But it can also be liberating, and fundamentally right and good.

Simply because curative treatment is no longer possible does not mean that doctors lose interest. Instead of concern about long-term side-effects of laxatives, for example, they are used in doses enough for relief. If breathing is becoming agitated or panicky, it may be reasonable to use doses of short-acting hypnotics – from the valium family – in order to comfort, even though normally there would be concern about addiction. Opiates are used in quantity and increased as need be. The 'double effect' is used: if pain is ongoing, opiates can be used in increasing quantity, even if this brings the side-effects of sedation, breathing decreasing and advancing death. We are now potential patients who are so squeamish about death that we have removed care of dying people from the normal repertoire of home, hearth and family doctors to regional hospices to deal with it for us. Certainly, many hospices offer excellent care for patients with specialist needs and who need constant nursing care. However, hospices are mainly run by charitable sector organisations and cannot guarantee to accept referrals. This means that some patients who wish to go into a hospice do not, and are instead admitted to hospital, or stay at home.

The patient paradox makes an appearance again. There will be some patients who will have a comfortable death at home, co-ordinated by the district nurses and GPs from the local surgery. If you have more difficult problems, which would need more nursing care, you had better hope that the lottery of hospice beds, or charitable sector palliative care nurses, can fill in the gaps. Why do we allow this? It would be fairer and kinder to everyone that the resource of end-of-life nursing was adequate for all who would benefit from it. District nurses, who had dealt with the dying since the beginning of the NHS, have become shadowed by the new breed of specialist nurse who deals only with terminal care. From being a core part of a nurse's workload, palliative care is now seen as something 'special', something distinct from usual nursing care. This has been mirrored in GPs' work, as we have deferred, perhaps too much, to hospices for caring for patients who could, given the right resources, have been cared for at home. Confidence comes with experience, reflection, and, for GPs, sharing and discussing care of patients within the practice. We are losing these skills.

There is always a role for improving knowledge and skills. GPs and patients will always benefit from having help from specialist doctors and nurses. However, district nurses and GPs have been moved from the centre to the periphery. Dying people must now rely on the generosity of strangers to fund overnight nursing care at home, or a place at a hospice. Should we not be doing much better than this? Don't dying patients deserve better?

The loss of 24-hour care

Sadly, the medical profession has been complicit in allowing the dissolution of the NHS. Part of the problem of providing continuity of care has been the loss of out-of-hours care responsibility by GPs. Before 2004, some GPs did their own out-of-hours work. If you were a GP in a remote or rural area, you could be on call for long stretches on your own. You would work daytime as well as nights. You relied on your patients – who would probably be well known to you – to call you only for genuine emergencies. In towns and cities, many GPs would work in groups to cover each other's patients at night. Two practices, making up eight doctors in all and covering a patient population, of, say, 10,000 patients, would each take a turn. Being constantly tired is draining and stressful. And not all calls to the out-of-hours service were urgent: people could call in about the best treatment for headlice, or about a rash that had been present for six months. Some patients complained that they could not get healthcare at a time that suited them. In an attempt to deal with the increased pressure on out-of-hours services, many parts of the country saw GPs pool together to set up community deputising centres, which could co-ordinate care between many practices, not just one or two. These could then designate GPs who assessed patients who could come to the centre, GPs who could travel to patients and GPs who would talk to patients on the telephone and advise them appropriately. They could filter out the non-urgent and try to concentrate on the sick.

The GP contract in 2004 allowed GPs to hand over out-of-hours care to primary care trusts (PCTs) and, with the financial gain of doing the out-of-hours being marginal, most did so. The calls to deal with the genuinely sick had become proportionately smaller. Providing decent palliative care was hard to do, since you were in a dimly lit bedroom, trying to set up a morphine pump and help a family's grief, all while answering your phone about other patients looking for more routine care. Most GPs did the sums, took a pay cut of about £6,000 and handed over the responsibility.[22]

The end result has been bad for patients. Doctors not familiar with the area – or even, in some cases, with the English language – flew in from Europe or elsewhere to deliver short term out-of-hours care. One man died after a German locum confused diamorphine dosages.[23] Private companies could tender for the work. Local GPs, either offered less pay or less control over their work, became less involved with private providers. In Cornwall, local GPs had provided care as an out-of-hours co-operative called KernowDoc. They addressed Parliament in 2004, saying that the shortfall in funding after the 2004 contract would 'be able to be made up by reconfiguring services, but this is not possible within the time scale for the opt-out. The PCTs will therefore either have to reduce the quality of the service, or find the difference from their base line, which is likely to affect other services.'[24] Serco, a private provider, then took over KernowDoc, supplying out-of-hours GP care. Responding to more than 80 complaints about the new service, a spokesman for the PCT who commissioned Serco said: 'It is a cheaper service than KernowDoc but I don't think that compromises quality.'[25] In 2006 an overseas doctor employed by Serco did not clinically assess an elderly man; responding to the complaint that was made, the director of Serco said the company would prefer to recruit local doctors to work there, but they were 'unable' to do so.[24]

There is no evidence that this new method of working has brought any benefits, and of course, if we do not look for harms, we will not find them. In Aberdeen, NHS 24 amended its telephone protocols after one teenager died of meningitis and a middle-aged man of septic shock after phoning for advice.[27] Another woman died as a consequence of diabetic coma, after phoning for telephone advice; at the inquest a consultant said: 'The telephone takes away the ability to spot if the patient is ill, which we rely on as a sixth sense rather than taking guidelines by rote.'[28] Yet people with minor symptoms were treated the same way as those with serious symptoms. It is hard to find one serious disease in a hundred, harder still to find it in ten thousand.

None of this is an argument against people seeking advice for minor illnesses. Instead, it is an argument that the NHS has ended up with a poor out-of-hours service because it has not prioritised the most sick. Instead, out-of-hours services were to be provided cheaply, and cheapness is no marker for quality.

Why medical professionalism matters

Doctors have a duty, first, to the patient. This is why medical school applicants are quizzed, at interview, about their motives. This is why medical students are taught ethics and it is why they must not have sexual or financial relationships with their patients. This is why the General Medical Council strikes doctors off its medical register for serious criminal convictions and why doctors must provide an address for registration where they are contactable by the GMC.

But these are coarse measures of professional practice. Doctors, for right or wrong, have power, and must not abuse this. When patients are unwell they become vulnerable – 'dissolving like a sugarcube' as Christopher Hitchens put it. It is not fair if doctors have to place other priorities, from contract blood pressure tickboxes to generating numbers for cervical screening, before their patients' needs.

It is dangerous when the 'care of the patient' is not the first concern of doctors. When doctors go by what governments tell them to do rather than what their professional code dictates, ghastliness ensues. This doesn't just happen in dictatorships abroad but in the UK. In the 1970s, doctors were employed by the Home Office in the UK to give immigrant women at Heathrow airport 'virginity tests', supposedly to satisfy visa requirements by proving they were not already married.[29] The medical records made by the doctors and kept on file, released in 2011, said that 'penetration of about half an inch made it apparent that she had an intact hymen'. Yet a non-intact hymen is not evidence of intercourse.[30] Doctors thus became complicit in facilitating a degrading and pointless examination. What 'care of the patient first' was evident there?

Or take Atos, a French electronics firm, which in 2005 won the contract to provide medical assessments for sickness benefits from the Department of Health. Part of the deal was that they must use GMC-registered doctors to do certain reports. The adverts to work for them, in the medical press, did not emphasise the qualities of the work, but the qualities outside of it. 'Getting home on time is part of my daily routine' says one.[31] Doctors can work for Atos either in a salaried role, or a sessional basis, where they are paid per case seen. All the doctors' work is audited, and the doctors are reprehended if they are not keeping up with the required number of assessments. The medical examination itself is based on a computer dropdown menu, which doctors have to tick off according to responses from the patient. Failing an assessment can mean that a person no longer receives benefits, which can have profound consequences.

Is the Atos assessment fair? If someone has a mental health problem, the doctor has to decide if the person is 'sweating and trembling'. This is a crude estimation of mental distress, and these are symptoms that medication would try to control. The assessment is done at a single point in time, and does not address conditions that fluctuate in severity, for example, rheumatoid arthritis, bipolar disorder, or chronic bronchitis.

At a recruitment evening I was told that we should not refer to the people attending for assessment as patients but 'claimants'. The Faculty of Occupational Medicine makes it clear that doctors providing advice on work should have the same professional standards as other doctors 'adequately assessing the patients' conditions, taking account of the history (including the symptoms, and the psychological and social factors), the patients' views, and where necessary examining the patient, providing or arranging advice, investigations or treatment where necessary.'[32] Professor Malcolm Harrington wrote, in an independent review of the Atos system:

> 'Some conditions are more subjective and evidently more difficult to assess. As a result some of the descriptors many not adequately reflect the full impact of such conditions on the individual's capacity for work. The final decision on assigning the claimant to one of the three categories theoretically rests with the Decision Maker at Jobcentre Plus but, in practice, the Atos assessment dominates the whole procedure. This imbalance needs correcting.'[33]

But how? Should doctors take part in a faulty assessment that may have detrimental effects on patients? The problem, to me, is that doctors are accepting work without having satisfied themselves that it is based in evidence and places 'care of the patient' first. In fact, the GMC argued this in a complaint against a doctor in 2010: its elected Investigation Committee decided that the doctor was not providing 'clinical care' because he was working for the Department of Work and Pensions.[34]

The act of doctors practising professionally without 'making the care of your patient your first concern' is of profound consequence. We can see that doctors could therefore take part in all kinds of acts: from taking court orders to dropping acid in the eyes of a convict in Iran, 'legally' blinding him; from providing venous routes to deliver fatal drugs on death row, to doing unreliable examinations for virginity.

What is medicine for? Paternalism has been twisted at its root. Historically, doctors have been rightly accused of not sharing or explaining enough of medicine so that patients, kept in the dark, have not been allowed to make their own good choices. But now doctors are seen as conduits to any demands, whether medically necessary or not. Cosmetic surgeons perform vulval reductions, penile enlargements or operations to give women unnaturally large breasts, no matter the risk that the patient has to take. When patients become customers, they lose the protection that proper medical professionalism should provide.

Doctors, for their own and their patients' sake, must reclaim professionalism and practice according to medical ethics and evidence, not fashion, not demand, not politics, not scaremongering. Doctors have, in a continual media battering post-Shipman, absorbed a guilt that has neither helped patients nor them to deliver better care. They have started to agree to anything, no matter how remote from true, powerful professionalism it may be. Medical vocation is sometimes seen as something embarrassing when it should be the crux on which good healthcare rests: the desire to do one's best, to practise medicine well and to put the care of the patient first.

The truly informed patient

Professional doctors should liberate patients. Patients should be able to expect fair information that enables them to make good choices about their health. Doctors who are free to act 'with the care of the patient as the first concern' would do this. It is likely, as we have discussed, that fully informed patients and doctors would choose to be screened less and may also choose fewer invasive procedures and fewer futile interventions at the end of life.

This is based in evidence. When politics start to come into play, decisions are taken out of the hands of doctors and patients and given to politicians and their management consultant friends instead. In 2008, £300 million was spent on management consultancy in the NHS.[35] For this money, the Department of Health received the advice that savings could be produced in the NHS by moving healthcare out of hospital and into the community, and doing fewer of what the consultancy calls 'procedures with limited clinical benefit'. This could be done, said McKinsey and Company, by 'providing decision aids'.[36] In fact, there were already plenty of indications for providing evidence-based and cost-effective medicine; but they had been largely ignored by politicians.

It's easy, especially for non-experts who are not aware of the depth and breadth of research findings and its limitations, to lift research evidence far out of context. One of the points McKinsey makes is that 'crisis resolution teams can reduce the need for admissions by 40-50% based on controlled trials'. In fact, it cites only one trial, which was published in the *BMJ* in 2005.[37] This study randomised patients to either home care from a crisis team or inpatient care in hospital. The results showed that a third of patients did not enter the trial, some because they were too ill and needed to be in hospital. For the remainder, a third in the experimental group, versus two-thirds in the inpatient care group, were admitted to hospital after six months. A quarter of the experimental group were admitted to a halfway 'crisis house' as opposed to a fifth of the hospital group. This is not quite the same victory for home care claimed by McKinsey.

Indeed, in the words of one patient, responding to the research:

'In a crisis, one has to pick up the phone. When one is unwell, the phone is the last thing one wants to use. . . In a crisis, one wants to feel safe. One does not feel safe in the community, in a crisis. One has to rely on one's family and friends to resolve the crisis . . . One is then refused access to a bed in a hospital . . . After the crisis has been resolved by one's family and friends, one is then subject to the humiliation of having had the crisis in full view of the local community . . . for whom is this service of benefit to please? I don't like it and they haven't really helped me much. Is it that it just aims to save the services money and keep people out of hospital?'[38]

It is one thing for a doctor to suggest treatment at home for a patient who would benefit from it and who would prefer it. It is quite another for a doctor to recommend it purely to save money at the behest of management consultants.

Or take another of McKinsey's suggestions, which was that 'decommissioning procedures with limited clinical benefit could drive savings of £0.3 – £0.7 billion across England'. One of the firm's tremendous ideas was to stop doing 'inguinal, umbilical and femoral hernias' because they are 'potentially cosmetic interventions'. These would be the same hernias that have a risk of strangulation, and which should be referred to hospital urgently, lest there be an intra-abdominal catastrophe.[39] Or what about their idea to stop doing 'minor skin surgery for non-cancer lesions' – an odd suggestion, since most skin lesions are diagnosed as cancer or not under a microscope, necessitating all suspicious lesions to be removed in the first place. Or the bizarre suggestion that cochlear implants do not need to be used in 'mild' cases, when only specialist centres fit these devices for people with specific types of severe deafness and after multidisciplinary assessment. McKinsey manages to muddle current practice with complex evidence – and patients are the losers. How on earth is a person with serious mental illness, in mid-crisis, meant to be able to work out if they are getting good advice to stay at home or not?

GP commissioning, as sought in England under the Coalition government, seriously threatens the relationship between patients and doctors. Previously, NICE sought to make judgments on the cost-effectiveness of interventions after a long period of researching the evidence, consulting with concerned groups, and careful statistical analysis. Rather than making NICE better – trying to remove as many conflicts of interest from members as possible, and being transparent about drug company costings, for example – its principles are being undermined. Judgments on cost-effectiveness will still have to be made but now by GP clinical commissioning groups. Not only is this inefficient, replicating work across the country, but it means potential inequalities. Rather than ensuring that everyone benefits from good interventions, the risk will increase of people not getting them because a local commissioning board says no. If your doctor denies you a treatment, will you, as a patient, feel confident that this is because it is an unsuitable treatment rather than an expensive one? NICE should be transparent, fair, and accountable. There is power, when acting on behalf of a whole health service, to tell manufacturers how much their price needs to be dropped by in order to make their drugs fairly cost-effective. The interface between doctors and patients has to be that of 'making the care of the patient the first concern'. GPs cannot have two conflicting masters: the patient and the Exchequer. Professional doctors who place patients first should, when they recommend a treatment or not, be trusted in their rationale.

Epilogue:

Why I am not a pessimist

The problem with writing a critical book is that the emphasis is not on a celebration of the qualities of evidence-based medicine and practice. The quiet side of medicine – avoiding the prescription of useless drugs, of supporting a person through to recovery from an episode of depression – has few ambassadors. Most media attention in healthcare is taken up with 'new' or 'breakthrough' treatments, which usually turn out to have been oversold or hyped. Yet the day-to-day business of doctoring is full of small significances, decisions and deliberations. These are the stitching through the fabric of professional, trusting relationships. The benefits of these interactions – concomitant professional outcomes – are intrinsically useful to patients. They also tend to be cost-effective, saving on unneeded hospital admissions and improving health outcomes. Yet doctors are locked into the politically set chasing of targets, and instructions to screen well people for disease. In the meantime other people have illnesses or potentially serious symptoms and become deprioritised in a healthcare system where shouting loudest, not needing most, is rewarded. This doesn't seem either equitable or useful. We overtreat the well and undertreat the sick. Everybody loses. Doctors become torn between their paymasters and their professional duties. People are lured to patienthood with snappy slogans and little Hippocratic pride. What's it all about?

The best preventive medicine is not delivered via cholesterol-lowering tablets; rather, it is delivered by paying attention to epidemiologists who consistently find that health inequalities worsen everyone's health. We should start believing the evidence enough to act on it. Reducing inequalities is where the biggest gains in health are to be made, not our current model of taking well people and screening them into diagnoses they don't need and won't benefit from. A politician a while ago decided that the NHS should stop being a 'national sickness service' – but that is what it needs to be. We have to stop discriminating against ill people. Sick people should get good healthcare. Preventing disease may sometimes be possible through medical action, but the biggest improvements to healthcare will be social and political. Anything else is nibbling at the edges, and averts our societial eye from the real problems, while we, deluded, start to believe our own medical hype.

There are improvements to healthcare that would be straightforward and are within our grasp. There is already an infrastructure of doctors who, in the main, trained out of vocation and want to treat patients, not accountancy balance sheets. Free them up to do so, audit and peer review them – professional pride is a strong medical trait, for everyone wants to be above average – and rather than chasing politically set targets, we can agree on evidence-based ones. The NHS could be made apolitical, running to the same method of NICE or SIGN, adopting evidence-based interventions and properly trialling ones that aren't. There is a role for the taxpayer and voter to decide how much they are willing to pay for a quality of life point as set by NICE; honest dialogue will help us get rid of the oversold and overhyped wares of healthcare marketeers. People should decide how much screening they wish to have, and ask more about the dilemmas and uncertainties they face before taking it up.

Knowledge is power, but we need knowledge, not hype, not misinformation, not sexed-up advertising slogans. Evidence needs to be imprinted in every medical decision we take, and that means no short-cut slogans. We need doctors to remain professionals, responsible in a way which is not subject to the fashions of healthcare charities, the influence of pharmaceutical companies, or the transience of party politics. I am optimistic because I think that doctors can do this, and want to do this. But the biggest push to better healthcare has to come from patients. For doctors to regain their professional upper hand, we need patients to demand something different. We all need a resurgence of medical professional values, and a rejection of the non-evidence-based initiatives and the flagrantly political stamping on the intimacy of our consultations. It is only with 'making the care of the patient the first concern' that the current patient paradox can be ended, the ill can be properly cared for and the well escape futile tests and treatment.

So, please, patients, help make the health service better. Hold us to account.

Glossary

Absolute risk A statistical way of representing risk: usually tells you what your chances are as a percentage. This method is distinct from relative risk. For example, reducing your risk from 2 in 100 to 1 in 100 is an expression of absolute risk. Although it's called 'risk', it really means chance. For example, the absolute risk, or chance, of a treatment being curative might be 5 in 100. Absolute risk is often contrasted with relative risk, see below. In the same examples, reducing an absolute risk from 2 in 100 to 1 in 100 is also a reduction in relative risk by 50%.

Bayesian A statistical method where a calculation of chance can be refined by the knowledge of new information.

Bias Bias can lead to trial results that are unlikely to be true or fair. There are different types of bias. Selection bias is when the people in the control group and intervention group taking part in a trial are not comparable, perhaps due to age, social class or sex. Attrition bias is when participants drop out of a study, perhaps due to side-effects, which may lead to the intervention appearing better than it actually is. High-quality studies reduce bias as much as possible.

Bipolar disorder Formally known as manic depression, this mood disorder results in abnormally high or low periods of mood. Bipolar 1 and 2 are further distinctions used in the US, with the difference being in the severity of high mood experienced.

Cancer Normally body cells live and die in a regulated way. Cancer results from cells that divide and grow in an unorganised way. Some cancers behave in a malignant manner, spreading and causing death. Other cancers are slow growing, or can be completely removed, or exist and cause few problems.

Cardiovascular risk This means the risk of heart attack, stroke, mini-stroke (TIA, or transient ischaemic attack), or angina. Cardiovascular disease can also lead to circulation problems, particularly in the feet or legs, and kidney disease as well as 'multi-infarct' dementia, where multiple mini-strokes cause memory loss. Contributions to cardiovascular risk include smoking, diabetes, high blood pressure, social deprivation, cholesterol and obesity.

Case control study This type of study is often used to study uncommon diseases. By matching a group of people with a disease to a group of very similar people without the disease, the groups can be compared to find other differences - like smoking or exposure to chemicals - between them. This type of study doesn't involve testing an intervention, such as a drug or other therapy.

Cervical smear A brush is used to take cells (take a 'smear') from the cervix, the neck of the womb, which are then examined microscopically. Some cellular changes may progress to cervical cancer, although most revert back to normal.

Cholesterol A fat essential in diet and which assists the absorption of fat-soluble vitamins. High levels in the blood are associated with increased cardiovascular risk. There are two components; HDL (high-density lipoprotein) and LDL (low density lipoprotein.) Lower cardiac risk is associated with high HDL levels, and higher cardiac risk with higher LDL levels.

Cohort study A group of people studied over time. This type of study observes people over time, rather than test an individual treatment or operation. Prospective rather than retrospective cohorts are more reliable.

Cochrane There are several organisations named after the British epidemiologist Archie Cochrane, all concerned with evidence in medicine. There is the Cochrane Review, which is a specifically organised systematic review of a given subject. The Cochrane Library is a collection of online review databases. The Cochrane Collaboration is the international organisation that organises and maintains systematic reviews. www. cochrane.org

Control group This group is used in a trial to compare the effects of a treatment or intervention. A control group informs about what would have happened without the treatment being tested. This is important because many conditions get better by themselves, over time. If a control group is not used, the researchers cannot be sure if it was the treatment, rather than chance or time, that led to any improvement in the study group.

Double blind Used to describe a trial where both the trial participant and the researcher do not know whether the placebo or active treatment is being used.

DCIS Ductal carcinoma in situ is a breast disorder usually found via X-ray at breast screening, which may go on to develop into an invasive cancer.

False negative A test gives a negative result when the person does have the disease or disorder being tested for.

False positive A test gives a positive result when the person does not have the disease or disorder being tested for.

Food and Drugs Administration (FDA) The Food and Drugs Administration is the US organisation responsible for ensuring the safety of medicines and medical devices. www.fda.gov

Framingham A town in Massachusetts, USA, which has run long-term studies of cardiovascular risk in its population since 1948. These data has informed most modern cardiovascular risk calculators. www. framinghamheartstudy.org

Herceptin The brand name for trastuzumab, a monoclonal antibody. This is one treatment used in HER-2 positive breast cancer, where HER-2 protein is present on the cancer cells. The drug acts as an antibody to the HER-2 proteins, stopping them from growing.

Intervention Used to describe many different types of healthcare, for example, physiotherapy, medicines, specially designed information leaflets, operations, or strength and balance training.

James Lind Library An online, free-to-access library about the history of fair tests of treatments at www.jameslindlibrary.org. James Lind was a physician who ran tests in 1747, showing that oranges and lemons were the best available treatments for scurvy.

Lifetime risk This is the chance of having a disease or disorder during a lifespan. For example, the lifetime risk of having breast cancer is now estimated at 1 in 8.

MHRA Medicines and Healthcare products Regulatory Agency. A UK governmental organisation responsible for ensuring that drugs and medical devices are effective and acceptably safe. www.mhra.gov.uk

Nocebo An intervention that has no biological effect but causes side-effects. For example, a person experiencing headaches after talking an inert tablet experiences a nocebo effect.

Number needed to treat (NNT) Number needed to treat is a means to convey how likely a benefit from an intervention is. For example, the NNT for middle ear infections with antibiotics in children is eight: for every one child who gets better faster with antibiotics, eight need to be treated. A similar means is used for number needed to screen: 2,000 women have to be breast screened over ten years in order to stop one death from breast cancer. A useful resource is www.thennt.com

p-values These are values attached to study results to denote degrees of certainty. High p-values denote less certainty about a finding, low values more certainty. A p-value of 0.05 means there is a one in 20 chance the findings are down to chance alone, and not the intervention being tested. A value of 0.05 or smaller is called 'statistically significant'. This particular value is simply convention and custom.

PHQ The Patient Health Questionnaire is a means of assessing the severity of depression. It is copyrighted to pharmaceutical company Pfizer.

Placebo Placebo describes a drug or treatment that does not have a biological effect. Placebo effects are the benefits observed in the patient when a placebo intervention is used.

Prostate Male gland that surrounds the neck of the bladder and tends to enlarge over time. A common site of cancers; some are aggressive, others are not.

Proxy outcomes Sometimes called surrogate outcomes. These are measurements that are not, by themselves, clinically useful, but are thought to be related to useful outcomes. For example, lowering blood pressure by itself is not the aim of treatment; rather, it is to lower the risk of later heart attack and stroke.

Randomised controlled trial (RCT) A group of similar people is randomly assigned to the intervention being tested, or the comparator(s). The comparator might be a placebo or the best current treatment. The difference between the groups is then compared. RCTs are favoured because they reduce bias and increase certainty.

Relative risk A measure of risk that is usually used to illustrate your increased or decreased risk with an intervention. Relative risk depends on what your risk was to start with. For example, a reduction in heart attacks with a treatment might reduce your risk by 50%, even if the risk was reduced by half, from 1 in 1,000 to 0.5 in 1,000. (see also Absolute risk)

Sensitivity How likely a test is to pick up a diagnosis. A sensitive test will pick up high numbers of people who have the disease being tested for.

Screening The act of looking for disease, disorder or risk in a person who is well and with no symptoms of disease.

Significance There are two main types; statistical significance and clinical significance. p-values of less than 0.05 are said to be statistically significant. However this does not mean a result is clinically significant, or useful. For example, a trial may show a drug has a p-value of 0.01 for being able to lower blood pressure. However, if this lowering is only 0.5mmHg, it is unlikely to be very useful for patients, and hence is not clinically significant.

Specificity How able a test is to correctly identify patients who do not have the disease being tested for. A highly specific test will identify high numbers of people who do not have the disease.

Statins A collection of drugs, including simvastatin, pravastatin and atorvastatin, usually taken daily, and which lower blood cholesterol levels.

Symptoms To have something noticeably different or wrong - for example, a cough, a rash, a headache, or a breast lump. Screening tests are not done in people with symptoms.

Systematic review A review of research literature that aims to answer a specific question by collecting, assessing and synthesising evidence. Only rarely is one research paper all that has been written on a subject. Systematic reviews aim to collate all available research and critically appraise it. Cochrane reviews, for example, follow a specific set of steps to prepare a review.

References

Chapter 1 To screen or not to screen – first do no harm

1. Wilson JM, Jungner G. *Principles and practices of screening for disease.* WHO, Geneva, 1968. whqlibdoc.who.int/php/WHO_PHP_34.pdf
2. Prescan. www.prescan.co.uk/
3. Lifescan. www.lifescanuk.org/
4. Welch, G. *Should I Be Tested for Cancer? Maybe not and here's why.* University of California Press. 2004
5. McCartney M. Executive health checks raise questions. *FT Magazine*, December 2008.
6. Vernooij MW, Arfan Ikram M. Incidental Findings on Brain MRI in the General Population. *N Engl J Med* 2007; 357:1821-1828 www.nejm.org/doi/full/10.1056/NEJMoa070972
7. Health Technology Assessment. Screening Programs for asymptomatic unruptured intracranial aneurysms: review of clinical effectiveness, cost-effectiveness, and evidence-based guidelines. *Canadian Agency for drugs and technologies in Health*, May 2010 www.cadth.ca/media/pdf/20100503-090753_l0173_screening_asymptomatic_aneurysms_final.pdf
8. International Study of Unruptured Intracranial Aneurysms: Unruptured Intracranial Aneurysms – Risk of Rupture and Risks of Surgical Intervention. *N Engl J Med* 1998; 339:1725-1733 www.nejm.org/doi/full/10.1056/NEJM199812103392401
9. BUPA Complete Health. www.bupa.co.uk/individuals/health-assessments/complete-health
10. Ottmar MD, Gonda RL Jr. Liver function tests in patients with computed tomography demonstrated hepatic metastases. *Gastrointest Radiol* 1989;14: 55-58 www.springerlink.com/content/x6kvhu744u700103/
11. Aragon G, Younossi ZM. When and how to evaluate mildly elevated liver enzymes in apparently healthy patients. *Cleve Clin J Med* 2010; 77:195-204. www.ccjm.org/content/77/3/195.long
12. Sibille M, Deigat N. Laboratory data in healthy volunteers: reference values, reference changes, screening and laboratory adverse event limits in Phase I clinical trials. *Eur J Clin Pharmacol* 1999; 55:13-9. www.ncbi.nlm.nih.gov/pubmed/10206079
13. Genetichealth 'Personal Health Management' website, accessed February 2011 www.genetic-health.co.uk/dna-test-services/premium-female.htm
14. Eeles RA, Stratton MR. The genetics of familial breast cancer and their practical implications. *Eur J Cancer* 1994; 30: 1383-90 www.sciencedirect.com/science/article/pii/0959804994901902
15. NICE. CG41: Familial breast cancer. London, 2006. www.nice.org.uk/nicemedia/pdf/CG41NICEguidance.pdf
16. Lord SJ, Lei W. A systematic review of the effectiveness of MRI as an addition to mammography and ultrasound in screening young women at high risk of breast cancer. *Eur J Cancer* 2007; 43: 1905-1917 www.ejcancer.info/article/S0959-8049(07)00484-4/abstract
17. Buys SS, Partridge E. The Prostate, Lung, Colorectal and Ovarian (PLCO) Cancer Screening Randomized Controlled Trial. *JAMA* 2011;305(22):2295-2303. jama.ama-assn.org/content/305/22/2295.long
18. UK Screening Portal, UK National Screening Committee, accessed February 2011 www.screening.nhs.uk/ovariancancer

19. Margolis J. The Interpretation of Genes. *Financial Times*, February 2009. www.genetic-health.co.uk/uploadfiles/FT10February2009.pdf

20. Clarke DM, Currie KC. Depression, anxiety and their relationship with chronic diseases: a review of the epidemiology, risk and treatment evidence. *Med J Australia* 2009; 190: S54–S60 www.mja.com.au/public/issues/190_07_060409/cla10974_fm.pdf

21. Scottish Intercollegiate Guidelines Network. SIGN 50: A guideline developer's handbook. Annex B: key to evidence statements and grades of recommendations. www.sign.ac.uk/guidelines/fulltext/50/annexb.html

22. More Doctors Smoke Camels Than Any Other Cigarette. 1949 Camel Cigarettes TV commercial. www.youtube.com/watch?v=gCMzjJjuxQI

23. Gardner MN, Brandt AM. "The doctors' choice is America's choice" The physician in US cigarette advertisements, 1930-1953. *Am J of Public Health* 2006; 96(2):222-232 ajph.aphapublications.org/doi/abs/10.2105/AJPH.2005.066654

24. Dobson R, Elliott J. Dr Spock's advice blamed for cot deaths. *The Times*, May 2005. www.timesonline.co.uk/tol/news/uk/health/article520623.ece (£)

25. Gilbert R, Salanti G, Harden M, See S. Infant sleeping position and the sudden infant death syndrome: systematic review of observational studies and historical review ofrecommendations from 1940 to 2002. *Int J Epidemio* 2005;34:874–887 ije.oxfordjournals.org/content/34/4/874.full.pdf

26. Hiley CM, Morley C. What do mothers remember about the 'back to sleep' campaign? *Arch Dis Child* 1995; 73: 496–497 www.ncbi.nlm.nih.gov/pmc/articles/PMC1511461/

27. Gilbert R, Salanti G. Infant sleeping position and the sudden infant death syndrome: systematic review of observational studies and historical review of recommendations from 1940 to 2002. *Int. J. Epidemiol* 2005 34: 874-887 ije.oxfordjournals.org/content/34/4/874.full

28. CRASH trial collaborators. Final results of MRC CRASH, a randomised placebo-controlled trial of intravenous corticosteroid in adults with head injury–outcomes at 6 months. *Lancet* 2005; 365: 1957-1959 www.thelancet.com/journals/lancet/article/PIIS0140-6736(05)66552-X/abstract

29. Sauerlanda S, Maegele M. A CRASH landing in severe head injury. *Lancet* 2004; 364: 1291-1292 www.thelancet.com/journals/lancet/article/PIIS0140-6736(04)17202-4/fulltext

30. Sanossian N, Arbi G. Frequency and Determinants of Nonpublication of Research in the Stroke Literature. *Stroke* 2006; 37: 2588-2592 stroke.ahajournals.org/content/37/10/2588.full

31. GlaxoSmithKline. Public disclosure of clinical research. Corporate Responsibility Report, 2010. www.gsk.com/responsibility/cr-report-2010/research-practices/public-disclosure-of-clinical-research/

32. Krall R, Rockhold F. More on compulsory registration of clinical trials: GSK has created useful register, *BMJ* 2005;330:479.3, 24th Febuary 2005 www.bmj.com/content/330/7489/479.3.full

33. Curfman GD, Morrissey S. Expression of Concern: Bombardier et al., "Comparison of Upper Gastrointestinal Toxicity of Rofecoxib and Naproxen in Patients with Rheumatoid Arthritis," *N Engl J Med* 2000; 343:1520-8. N Engl J Med, online editorial, December 2008. www.nejm.org/doi/full/10.1056/NEJMe058314

Chapter 2 The business of cardiovascular risk

1. UK election: the main parties' health policies. *Lancet*, 375, 9725, 1511-1514, 1 May 2010 www.thelancet.com/journals/lancet/article/PIIS0140-6736(10)60642-3/fulltext

2. The Scottish Government: Universal health checks planned. March 2010 www. scotland.gov.uk/News/Releases/2010/03/22081937

3. NHS Choices website, NHS Health Check, accessed February 2011 http://www.nhs. uk/Planners/NHSHealthCheck/Pages/NHSHealthCheckandyou.aspx

4. NHS The Information Centre. Prescriptions Dispensed in the Community: England, Statistics for 1999 to 2009 Information Centre www.ic.nhs.uk/webfiles/publications/ prescriptionsdispensed/Prescriptions_Dispensed_1999_2009%20.pdf

5. Cholesterol Treatment Trialists' Collaborators. Efficacy and safety of cholesterol-lowering treatment: prospective meta-analysis of data from 90 056 participants in 14 randomised trials of statins. The Lancet; 366: 1267-1278 www.thelancet.com/journals/ lancet/article/PIIS0140-6736(05)67394-1/abstract

6. Thavendiranathan P, Bagai A. Primary Prevention of Cardiovascular Diseases with Statin Therapy. *Arch Intern Med* 2006; 166: 2307-2313 archinte.ama-assn.org/cgi/ content/full/166/21/2307

7. Graham DJ, Staffa JA. Incidence of hospitalized rhabdomyolysis in patients treated with lipid-lowering drugs. *JAMA* 2004 Dec 1;292(21):2585-90. Epub 2004 Nov 22.

8. Sattar N, Preiss D. Statins and risk of incident diabetes: a collaborative meta-analysis of randomised statin trials. *Lancet*; 375: 735–742 www.thelancet.com/journals/lancet/ article/PIIS0140-6736(09)61965-6/abstract

9. Wenger NK. Preventing cardiovascular disease in women: an update. *Clin Cardiol* 2008; 31:109-13. onlinelibrary.wiley.com/doi/10.1002/clc.20134/abstract

10. Abramson J, Wright JM. Are lipid-lowering guidelines evidence-based? *Lancet*; 369: 168 -169 www.thelancet.com/journals/lancet/article/PIIS0140-6736(07)60084-1/ fulltext

11. Samia M, Glynn RJ. Trials. Statins for the Primary Prevention of Cardiovascular Events in Women With Elevated High-Sensitivity C-Reactive Protein or Dyslipidaemia: Results From the Justification for the Use of Statins in Prevention: An Intervention Trial Evaluating Rosuvastatin (JUPITER) and Meta-Analysis of Women From Primary Prevention Trials. *Circulation*; 2010: 1069-1077) circ.ahajournals.org/ content/121/9/1069

12. Ford I, Murray H. Long-Term Follow-up of the West of Scotland Coronary Prevention Study. *N Engl J Med* 2007; 357:1477-1486 www.nejm.org/doi/full/10.1056/ NEJMoa065994#t=articleTop

13. Heart Protection Study Collaborative Group, *Lancet*, 378;9808:2013–2020

14. British Hypertension Society working party. Treating mild hypertension. *BMJ* 1989; 298: 694-698 www.ncbi.nlm.nih.gov/pmc/articles/PMC1836038/

15. Sever P, Beevers G. Management guidelines in essential hypertension: report of the second working party of the British Hypertension Society. *BMJ* 1993; 306: 983-987 www.ncbi.nlm.nih.gov/pmc/articles/PMC1677457/pdf/bmj00015-0045.pdf

16. Ramsay LE, Williams B. British Hypertension Society guidelines for hypertension management 1999: summary. *BMJ* 1999; 319: 630 www.bmj.com/ content/319/7210/630.full

17. Williams B, Poulter NR. British Hypertension Society guidelines for hypertension management 2004 (BHS-IV): summary. *BMJ* 2004; 328: 634 www.bmj.com/content/3 28/7440/634?view=long&pmid=15016698

18. NICE. CG127: Clinical management of primary hypertension in adults. London, 2011. www.nice.org.uk/nicemedia/live/13561/56008/56008.pdf

19. Wright JM, Musini VM. First-line drugs for hypertension. *Cochrane Database Syst Rev.* 2009; 3: CD001841 onlinelibrary.wiley.com/doi/10.1002/14651858.CD001841.

pub2/abstract

20. Quan A, Kerlikowske K. Pharmacotherapy for hypertension in women of different races. *Cochrane Database Syst Rev.* 2000; 3: CD002146. onlinelibrary.wiley.com/doi/10.1002/14651858.CD002146/abstract

21. Musini VM,Tejani AM. Pharmacotherapy for hypertension in the elderly. *Cochrane Database Syst Rev.* 2009; 4: CD000028 onlinelibrary.wiley.com/doi/10.1002/14651858.CD000028.pub2/abstract

22. Cranney M, Warren E. Hypertension in the elderly: attitudes of British patients and general practitioners. *J Hum Hypertens* 1998; 12: 539–545 www.nature.com/jhh/journal/v12/n8/pdf/1000656a.pdf

23. General Medical Council. Good Medical Practice: Providing good clinical care. www.gmc-uk.org/guidance/good_medical_practice/good_clinical_care_index.asp

Chapter 3 The nature of cancer: breast beating

1. McFarlane MJ, Feinstein AR. The 'Epidemiologic Necropsy'. Unexpected Detections, Demographic Selections, and Changing Rates of Lung Cancer. *JAMA*.1987; 258:331-338 jama.ama-assn.org/content/258/3/331.abstract

2. Sens MA, Zhou X. Unexpected neoplasia in autopsies: potential implications for tissue and organ safety. *Arch Pathol Lab Med.* 2009;133:1923-31. www.archivesofpathology.org/doi/full/10.1043/1543-2165-133.12.1923

3. Veress B, Alafuzoff I. A retrospective analysis of clinical diagnoses and autopsy findings in 3,042 cases during two different time periods. *Hum Pathol.* 1994; 25:140-5. www.sciencedirect.com/science/article/pii/0046817794902690

4. Ernster VL, Ballard-Barbash R. Detection of Ductal Carcinoma in Situ in Women Undergoing Screening Mammography. *J Natl Cancer Inst* 2002; 94: 1546-1554. jnci.oxfordjournals.org/content/94/20/1546.long

5. NHS Breast Screening Programme. Overcoming Barriers - Annual Review 2010. www.cancerscreening.nhs.uk/breastscreen/publications/nhsbsp-annualreview2010.pdf

6. Sanders ME, Schuyler PA. The natural history of low-grade ductal carcinoma in situ of the breast in women treated by biopsy only revealed over 30 years of long-term follow-up. *Cancer* 2005; 103: 2481-2484 onlinelibrary.wiley.com/doi/10.1002/cncr.21069/abstract

7. Virnig BA, Tuttle TM. Ductal carcinoma in situ of the breast: A systematic review of incidence, treatment, and outcomes. *J Natl Cancer Inst* 2010; 102(3):170-178 jnci.oxfordjournals.org/content/102/3/170.long

8. Welch HG, Black WC. Using Autopsy Series To Estimate the Disease "Reservoir" for Ductal Carcinoma in Situ of the Breast: How Much More Breast Cancer Can We Find? *Ann Intern Med* 1997; 127: 1023-1028 www.annals.org/content/127/11/1023.abstract

9. Dixon JM. Breast screening has increased the number of mastectomies. *Breast Cancer Research* 2009, 11(Suppl 3):S19 breast-cancer-research.com/content/11/S3/S19

10. Flanders J. Reality of ductal carcinoma in situ. *BMJ* 2009; 338:b958 www.bmj.com/content/338/bmj.b958

11. Conservative Party. The next moves forward. 1987 www.conservativemanifesto.com/1987/1987-conservative-manifesto.shtml

12. Currie E. *Life Lines.* London: Sidgwick and Jackson, 1989

13. NHS Breast Screening. Department of Health 2011. www.cancerscreening.nhs.uk/breastscreen/publications/nhsbsp.pdf

14. Advisory Committee on Breast Cancer Screening. Screening for breast cancer

in England: past and future. *J Med Screen* 2006;13:59–61 jms.rsmjournals.com/content/13/2/59.full.pdf

15. Advisory Committee on Breast Cancer Screening. Screening for breast cancer in England: past and future. *NHSBSP Publication* No 61, 2006 www.cancerscreening.nhs.uk/breastscreen/publications/nhsbsp61.pdf

16. International Agency for Research on Cancer. *IARC Handbook of Cancer Prevention Volume 7: Breast Cancer Screening*, Chapter 5: Effectiveness of screening. IARC Press, Lyon 2002. www.iarc.fr/en/publications/pdfs-online/prev/handbook7/Handbook7_Breast-5.pdf

17. Gøtzsche PC, Nielsen M. Screening for breast cancer with mammography. *Cochrane Database Syst Rev* 2011, Issue 1. Art. No.: CD001877. DOI: 10.1002/14651858. CD001877.pub4. onlinelibrary.wiley.com/doi/10.1002/14651858.CD001877.pub4/pdf

18. Nordic Cochrane Centre, 2012 'What you always wanted to know about breast screening' Accessed February 2012 www.cochrane.dk/screening/mammography-leaflet.pdf

19. Advisory Committee on Breast Cancer Screening. Screening for Breast Cancer in England: Past and Future. *NHSBSP Publication* No 61, February 2006 www.cancerscreening.nhs.uk/breastscreen/publications/nhsbsp61.pdf

20. Yaffe MJ, Mainprize JG. Risk of Radiation-induced Breast Cancer from Mammographic Screening. *Radiology* 2011; 258: 98-105 radiology.rsna.org/content/258/1/98.abstract

21. Loughran CF, Keeling C. Seeding of tumour cells following breast biopsy: a literature review. *Breast Cancer Research* 2010; 12(Suppl 3): 43 breast-cancer-research.com/content/12/S3/P43

Chapter 4 Smears and fears: the Jade Goody effect

1. Weaver M. Tributes pour in for Jade Goody after reality star dies from cancer, aged 27. *Guardian*, March 2009 www.guardian.co.uk/media/2009/mar/22/jade-goody-dies-tributes

2. Cancer Research UK. Preventing cervical cancer. April 2004 www2.units.it/brancaleone/leaflet_cervical_apr04.pdf

3. NHS Scotland. The Cervical Screening Test. Put it on Your List. 2010 www.healthscotland.com/uploads/documents/13485-TheCervicalScreeningTest.pdf

4. Raffle AE, Alden B. Outcomes of screening to prevent cancer: analysis of cumulative incidence of cervical abnormality and modelling of cases and deaths prevented. *BMJ* 2003; 326 : 901 www.ncbi.nlm.nih.gov/pmc/articles/PMC153831/

5. Crane JM. Pregnancy outcome after loop electrosurgical excision procedure: a systematic review. *Obstet Gynecol.* 2003;102: 1058-62. www.sciencedirect.com/science/article/pii/S0029784403007415

6. Samson SL, Bentley JR. The effect of loop electrosurgical excision procedure on future pregnancy outcome. *Obstet Gynecol.* 2005;105: 325-32. journals.lww.com/greenjournal/Abstract/2005/02000/The_Effect_of_Loop_Electrosurgical_Excision.19.aspx

7. Cancer Research UK. Cervical cancer statistics-UK info.cancerresearchuk.org/cancerstats/types/cervix/incidence/

8. Office of National Statistics. Cancer Trends in England and Wales, 1950-1999, Chapter 6 http://www.ons.gov.uk/ons/rel/cancer-unit/cancer-trends-in-england-and-wales/smps-no--66/index.html

9. Papanicolaou GN, Traut HF. *Diagnosis of uterine cancer by vaginal smear*. Oxford:

Commonwealth Fund, Oxford University, 1943.

10. Lund, CJ. An Epitaph for Cervical Carcinoma. *JAMA*. 1961;175(2):98-99 jama.ama-assn.org/content/175/2/98.abstract

11. Debates about cervical screening: an historical overview. *J Epidemiol Community Health* 2008; 62:284-287 jech.bmj.com/content/62/4/284.extract

12. Clarke EA, Anderson TW. Does screening by 'PAP' smears help prevent cervical cancer? A Case-control Study. *Lancet*. 1979; 314: 8132. www.ncbi.nlm.nih.gov/pubmed/87887

13. Apostolides A, Henderson M. Evaluation of Cancer Screening Programs. Parallels with Clinical Trials. *Cancer* 1977; 39:1779-1785. onlinelibrary.wiley.com/doi/10.1002/1097-0142(197704)39:4%2B%3C1779::AID-CNCR2820390805%3E3.0.CO;2-9/pdf

14. Peto J, Gilham C. The cervical cancer epidemic that screening has prevented in the UK. *Lancet* 2004; 364, 249 – 256 www.thelancet.com/journals/lancet/article/PIIS0140-6736(04)16674-9/fulltext

15. NHS Cervical Screening Programme. Cervical screening saves thousands of lives. July 2004 cancerscreening.nhs.uk/cervical/news/010.html

16. Modernising the NHSCSP: Introduction of LBC and change in national policy, NHS Cervical Screening Programme, 22/10/03 cancerscreening.nhs.uk/cervical/news/009.html

17. Jacobs K. Why should we be refused a smear test? *Guardian*; March 2009 www.guardian.co.uk/commentisfree/2009/mar/05/health-health

18. Marie Stopes International. Marie Stopes International welcomes government review of the UK's cervical screening policy. March 2009 www.mariestopes.org.uk/PressReleases/UK/Marie_Stopes_International_welcomes_government_review_of_the_UK%E2%80%99s_cervical_screening_policy.aspx

19. Advisory Committee on Cervical Screening. Extraordinary Meeting to re-examine current policy on cervical screening for women aged 20-24 years taking account of any new evidence and to make recommendations to the National Cancer Director and Ministers. May 2009 www.cancerscreening.nhs.uk/cervical/cervical-review-minutes-20090519.pdf

20. Simsir A, Brooks S. Cervicovaginal smear abnormalities in sexually active adolescents. Implications for management. *Acta Cytol*. 2002; 46:271-6. www.acta-cytol.com/toc/auto_abstract.php?id=16049

21. Robertson JH, Woodend BE. Risk of cervical cancer associated with mild dyskaryosis *BMJ* 1988; 297: 18-21 www.bmj.com/content/297/6640/18.short

22. Sasieni P, Castanon A. Effectiveness of cervical screening with age: population based case-control study of prospectively recorded data. *BMJ* 2009; 339:b2968 www.bmj.com/content/339/bmj.b2968

Chapter 5 Screening for more: the prostate, bowel and aorta

1. Abbasi K. To screen or not to screen? BMJ 1998; 316 : 484 www.bmj.com/content/316/7129/484.full

2. Thompson IM, Ankherst DP. Prostate-specific antigen in the early detection of prostate cancer. CMAJ 2007; 176: 1853-1858 www.cmaj.ca/content/176/13/1853.full

3. Ablin RJ. The Great Prostate Mistake. New York Times, March 2010. www.nytimes.com/2010/03/10/opinion/10Ablin.html

4. Lefevre ML. Prostate Cancer Screening: More Harm Than Good? *Am Fam Physician* 1998 Aug 1;58(2):432-438 www.aafp.org/afp/1998/0801/p432.html

5. Schröder FH, Hugosson J. Screening and Prostate-Cancer Mortality in a Randomized

European Study. *N Engl J Med* 2009; 360:1320-1328 www.nejm.org/doi/full/10.1056/NEJMoa0810084

6. Andriole GL, Crawford ED. Mortality Results from a Randomized Prostate-Cancer Screening Trial. *N Engl J Med* 2009; 360:1310-1319 www.nejm.org/doi/full/10.1056/NEJMoa0810696

7. Lin K, Lipsitz R. *Benefits and Harms of Prostate-Specific Antigen Screening for Prostate Cancer.* Agency for Healthcare Research and Quality (US), August 2008. www.annals.org/content/149/3/192.abstract

8. Barry MJ. Early Detection and Aggressive Treatment of Prostate Cancer. *J Gen Intern Med* 2000; 15: 749–751 www.ncbi.nlm.nih.gov/pmc/articles/PMC1495598/

9. Barry MJ, Mulley Jr AJ. Why Are a High Overdiagnosis Probability and a Long Lead Time for Prostate Cancer Screening So Important? *J Natl Cancer Inst* 2009; 101: 374-383. jnci.oxfordjournals.org/content/101/6/362.long

10. Stamey TA, Yang N. Prostate-Specific Antigen as a Serum Marker for Adenocarcinoma of the Prostate. *N Engl J Med* 1987; 317:909-916 www.nejm.org/doi/full/10.1056/NEJM198710083171501

11. Baker B. Medicare's new PSA coverage, revised CPT lab panels. *ACP–ASIM Observer*, February 2000 www.acpinternist.org/archives/2000/02/qanda.htm

12. Melia J, Moss S. Survey of the rate of PSA testing in general practice. *Brit J Cancer* 2001; 85; 656–657 www.ncbi.nlm.nih.gov/pmc/articles/PMC2364127/pdf/85-6691962a.pdf

13. Franks LM, Latent Carcinoma of the Prostate, *J Pathol Bacteriol*, 68,2,603-606.

14. Baker M, Standford Report, 22/9/04 Common test for prostate cancer comes under fire news.stanford.edu/news/2004/september22/med-prostate-922.html

15. Stamey TA, Caldwell M. The Prostate Specific Antigen Era in the United States is over for Prostate Cancer: What Happened in the Last 20 Years? *J Urol*, 172: 1297-1301 www.jurology.com/article/S0022-5347(05)61155-X/abstract

16. Rich AR, On the frequency of occurance of occult carcinoma of the prostate. *The Journal of Urology, 33:3 1935.* ije.oxfordjournals.org/content/36/2/274.full.pdf+html

17. A Tale of Two Brothers. The Prostate Centre, London, 2011 www.theprostatecentre.com/prostate-centre-patients/patient-stories/a-tale-of-two-brothers

18. NHS Bowel Cancer Screening Pilot, 2007. www.cancerscreening.nhs.uk/bowel/pilot.html

19. NHS Cancer Screening Programmes Bowel Cancer Screening. The colonoscopy Investigation www.cancerscreening.nhs.uk/bowel/publications/colonoscopy-investigation.pdf

20. Hewitson P, Glasziou P. Screening for colorectal cancer using the faecal occult blood test, Hemoccult. 2008, John Wiley & Sons onlinelibrary.wiley.com/doi/10.1002/14651858.CD001216.pub2/abstract

21. The NHS Abdominal Aortic Aneurysm Screening Programme. Information for Healthcare Professionals. aaa.screening.nhs.uk/professionals

22. Thompson SG, Ashton HA. Screening men for abdominal aortic aneurysm: 10 year mortality and cost effectiveness results from the randomised Multicentre Aneurysm Screening Study. *BMJ* 2009; 338:b2307 www.bmj.com/content/338/bmj.b2307?view=long&pmid=19553269

23. Schlösser FJ, Vaartjes I. Mortality after elective abdominal aortic aneurysm repair. *Ann Surg* 2010;251:158-64. journals.lww.com/annalsofsurgery/Abstract/2010/01000/Mortality_After_Elective_Abdominal_Aortic_Aneurysm.24.aspx

24. Irvine CD, Shaw E. A Comparison of the Mortality Rate After Elective Repair of

Aortic Aneurysms Detected Either by Screening or Incidentally. *Eur J Vasc Endovasc Surg*; 20: 374-378 www.sciencedirect.com/science/article/pii/S1078588400911870

25. Beck AW, Goodney PP. Predicting 1-year mortality after elective abdominal aortic aneurysm repair, *J Vasc Surg* 49;4:838-844, April 2009 http://www.jvascsurg.org/article/S0741-5214(08)01880-6/abstract

26. Khaira HS, Herbert LM. Screening for abdominal aortic aneurysms does not increase psychological morbidity. *Ann R Coll Surg Engl* 1998; 80: 341–342 www.ncbi.nlm.nih.gov/pmc/articles/PMC2503123/?page=1

27. Lifeline Screening. Screening for abdominal aortic aneurysm. www.lifelinescreening.co.uk/health-screening-services/abdominal-aortic-aneurysm.aspx

Chapter 6 Health for sale: everyone wants a slice of the healthy patient

1. Hope J. Low-cholesterol spread 'not certain to cut heart risks', GPs told. *Daily Mail*, May 2008. www.dailymail.co.uk/health/article-1023212/Low-cholesterol-spread-certain-cut-heart-risks-GPs-told.html

2. Florahearts.co.uk. Frequently asked questions. www.flora-professional.co.uk/plant_sterols.asp

3. Shepherd J, Cobbe SM. Prevention of coronary heart disease with pravastatin in men with hypercholesterolemia. *New Eng J Med* 1995; 333: 1301-1307 www.nejm.org/doi/full/10.1056/NEJM199511163332001

4. www.framinghamheartstudy.org/

5. Randomised trial of cholesterol lowering in 4444 patients with coronary heart disease: the Scandinavian Simvastatin Survival Study (4S). *Lancet* 1994; 344:1383-9. www.thelancet.com/journals/lancet/article/PIIS0140-6736(94)90566-5/abstract

6. Flora pro-activ. Lowering your Cholesterol, September 2009. 162.61.226.126/pdf/Lowering%20Your%20Cholesterol.pdf

7. Flora pro-activ. Plant Sterols Scientific Review, June 2009. www.flora-professional.co.uk www.flora-professional.co.uk/pdf/The%20science%20behind%20plant%20sterols_Scientific%20reviews%20(long%20version).pdf

8. Danone. What is Activia? www.activia.ie www.activia.ie/index.php/activia-explained/what-is-activia/5

9. Probiotics in Practice. www.probioticsinpractice.co.uk/introduction-to-probiotics.aspx

10. Danone Research. Clinical Studies. www.studies.danone.com/

11. Guyonneta D, Schlumberger A. Fermented milk containing Bifidobacterium lactis DN-173 010 improves gastrointestinal well-being and digestive symptoms in women reporting minor digestive symptoms: a randomised, double-blind, parallel, controlled study. *Br J Nutrition* 2009; 102: 1654-1662 journals.cambridge.org/action/displayAbstract?fromPage=online&aid=6731400

12. Guyonnet D, Woodcock A. Fermented milk containing Bifidobacterium lactis DN-173 010 improved self-reported digestive comfort amongst a general population of adults. A randomized, open-label, controlled, pilot study. *J Digestive Diseases* 2009; 10: 61-70 onlinelibrary.wiley.com/doi/10.1111/j.1751-2980.2008.00366.x/abstract

13. Agrawal A, Houghton LA. Clinical trial: the effects of a fermented milk product containing Bifidobacterium lactis DN-173 010 on abdominal distension and gastrointestinal transit in irritable bowel syndrome with constipation. Alimentary Pharmacology & Therapeutics 2009; 29:104–114. onlinelibrary.wiley.com/doi/10.1111/j.1365-2036.2008.03853.x/abstract

14. Guyonnet D, Chassany O. Effect of a fermented milk containing Bifidobacterium

animalis DN-173 010 on the health-related quality of life and symptoms in irritable bowel syndrome in adults in primary care: a multicentre, randomized, double-blind, controlled trial. Alimentary Pharmacology & Therapeutics 2007; 26:475–486. onlinelibrary.wiley.com/doi/10.1111/j.1365-2036.2007.03362.x/abstract

15. Advertising Standards Authority. ASA Adjudication on Coca-Cola Great Britain, October 2009. www.asa.org.uk/ASA-action/Adjudications/2009/10/Coca_Cola-Great-Britain/TF_ADJ_47037.aspx

16. De-Regil LM, Fernández-Gaxiola AC. Effects and safety of periconceptional folate supplementation for preventing birth defects. *Cochrane Database Syst Rev*. 2011; 10: CD007950 onlinelibrary.wiley.com/doi/10.1002/14651858.CD007950.pub2/pdf

17. Irlam JH, Visser MME. Micronutrient supplementation in children and adults with HIV infection. *Cochrane Database Syst Rev*. 2010; 12: CD003650 apps.who.int/rhl/reviews/CD003650.pdf

18. Caraballoso M, Sacristan M. Drugs for preventing lung cancer in healthy people. *Cochrane Database Syst Rev*. 2003; 2: CD002141 onlinelibrary.wiley.com/doi/10.1002/14651858.CD002141/pdf

19. Bjelakovic G, Nikolova N. Antioxidant supplements for prevention of mortality in healthy participants and patients with various diseases. *Cochrane Database Syst Rev*. 2008; 2: CD007176 onlinelibrary.wiley.com/doi/10.1002/14651858.CD007176/pdf/standard

20. Mishell DR. Goodwin TM, Brenner PF. Management of common problems in obstetrics and gynecology (fourth edition), Blackwell 2002

21. Babystart Pre-conception fertility fertilityshop.com/shop/index.php?main_page=product_info&cPath=1&products_id=15

22. Aboulghar MA, Mansour RT. Diagnosis and management of unexplained infertility: an update. *Arch Gynecol Obstet* 2003; 267:177-188 www.springerlink.com/content/6bfr0hc8kngget8f/

23. Guzick DS, Overstreet JW. Sperm morphology, motility and concentration in fertile and infertile men. N Engl J Med 2001; 345:1388-1393 www.nejm.org/doi/full/10.1056/NEJMoa003005#t=articleDiscussion

24. Zita West www.zitawest.com/about-zita-west-fertility-clinic/

25. The Zita West Fertility MOT www.zitawest.com/buy/services/tests/fertility-mot-amh-diy-test-kit.htm.htm

26. *Reproductive Ageing*. Royal College of Obstetricians and Gynaecologists, 2010

27. Nuffield Health, Fertility MOT, accessed Feburary 2012 www.nuffieldhealth.com/treatments/fertility-mot

28. Ritchie G. Fertility MOT made wannabe mum realise she had to get a move on if she wanted to conceive. *The Daily Record*, Jun 2010. www.dailyrecord.co.uk/news/real-life/2010/06/04/fertility-mot-made-wannabe-mum-realise-she-had-to-get-a-mo

29. Boots. Cervical Cancer Vaccination. www.boots.com/en/Cervical-Cancer-Vaccination_1150826/

30. ASCCP. Practice Management. Natural History of HPV www.asccp.org/practicemanagement/hpv/naturalhistoryofhpv/tabid/5962/default.aspx

31. Paavonen J, Naud P. Efficacy of human papillomavirus (HPV)-16/18 AS04-adjuvanted vaccine against cervical infection and precancer caused by oncogenic HPV types (PATRICIA): final analysis of a double-blind, randomised study in young women. Lancet 2009; 374: 301–314 www.thelancet.com/journals/lancet/article/PIIS0140-6736(09)61248-4/fulltext

32. FUTURE II Study Group. Quadrivalent Vaccine against Human Papillomavirus to

Prevent High-Grade Cervical Lesions. *N Engl J Med* 2007; 356:1915-1927 www.nejm.org/doi/full/10.1056/NEJMoa061741

33. Sigurdsson R, Briem H. The efficacy of HPV 16/18 vaccines on sexually active 18–23 year old women and the impact of HPV vaccination on organized cervical cancer screening. *Acta Obstetrica et Gynecologica Scandinavia*, 2009, Vol 8, Pages 27-35 informahealthcare.com/doi/abs/10.1080/00016340802566770

Chapter 7 George Clooney and the medical certainty illusion

1   Rorke B, Pathologic diagnosis as the gold standard. *Cancer.* 1997 Feb 15;79(4):665-7. www.ncbi.nlm.nih.gov/pubmed/9024702

2. Presant CA, Russell WO, Alexander RW, Fu YS. Soft-tissue and bone sarcoma histopathology peer review: the frequency of disagreement in diagnosis and the need for second pathology opinions. The Southeastern Cancer Study Group experience. *J Clin Oncol* 1986; 4:1658 – 1661 jco.ascopubs.org/content/4/11/1658.abstract

3. Baak JPA, Lindeman J, Overdiep SH, Langley FA. Disagreement of histopathological diagnoses of different pathologists in ovarian tumors – with some theoretical considerations. *Eur J Obstet Gyn R B* 1982; 13(1):51-55. www.sciencedirect.com/science/article/pii/0028224382900375

4. Farmer ER, Gonin, R, Hanna MP. Discordance in the histopathologic diagnosis of melanoma and melanocytic nevi between expert pathologists. *Hum Pathol.* 1996; 27(6): 528-531 www.ncbi.nlm.nih.gov/pubmed/8666360

5. Swerlick RA, Solomon ARR. Clinical diagnosis of moles vs Melanoma. *JAMA* 1998; 280(10):881-882 jama.ama-assn.org/content/280/10/881.extract

6. Vishal, K. *Frequency and clinical importance of pathological discordance in lymphoma.* University of Toronto 2009; 151 https://tspace.library.utoronto.ca/bitstream/1807/18799/6/Kukreti_Vishal_200911_MSc_thesis.pdf

7. Gill C, Sabin L. Why clinicians are natural Bayesians. *BMJ* 2005; 330:1080 www.bmj.com/content/330/7499/1080.extract

8. Morris AH. Developing and implementing computerized protocols for standardization of clinical decisions. *Ann Intern Med* 2000; 132(5):373-383 www.annals.org/content/132/5/373.abstract

9. Garg AX, Adhikari NK. Effects of computerized clinical decision support systems on practitioner performance and patient outcomes. *JAMA* 2005; 293(10):1223-1238 jama.ama-assn.org/content/293/10/1223.short

Chapter 8 The snowballing of protocols

1. Morrell CJ, Munro J.Impact of NHS Direct on other services: the characteristics and origins of its nurses. *Emerg Med J* 2002; 19:337-340 emj.bmj.com/content/19/4/337.long

2. Munro J, Nicholl J. Evaluation of NHS Direct first wave sites. First interim report to the Department of Health, University of Sheffield 1998 www.shef.ac.uk/polopoly_fs/1.43643!/file/nhsd1.pdf

3. Dealing with a patient who has a 10-year smear gap. Pulse Today. November 2011 www.pulsetoday.co.uk/main-content/-/article_display_list/10874619/www.pulsetoday.co.uk/main-content/-/article_display_list/10874619/dealing-with-a-patient-who-has-a-10-year-smear-gap

4. Uitti RJ, Calne DB, Dickson DW, Wszolek ZK. Is the neuropathological 'gold-standard' diagnosis dead? Implications of clinicopathological findings in an autosomal dominant neurodegenerative disorder. *Parkinsonism & Related Disorders* 2004;

   10(8):461-463

5. Rivett G, How is General Practice funded? www.nhshistory.net/gppay.pdf

6. Parker G. Is depression overdiagnosed? Yes. *BMJ*, 2007;335:328 August 2007. www.bmj.com/content/335/7615/328.full

7. Healy D. *The anti-depressant era*. Cambridge, MA: Harvard University Press,1997.

8. The NHS Information Centre Prescribing Support Unit. Prescriptions dispensed in the community, statistics for 1999 to 2009: England. The Health and Social Care Information Centre, 2010. www.ic.nhs.uk/

9. Coyne JC, Schwenk TL. The relationship of distress to mood disturbance in primary care and psychiatric populations. *J Consult Clin Psychol* 1997; 65(1):161-168 psycnet.apa.org/journals/ccp/65/1/161/

10. Kessler D, Bennewith O. Detection of depression and anxiety in primary care: follow up study. *BMJ* 2002; 325(7371):1016-1017 www.bmj.com/content/325/7371/1016.1.full.pdf

11. Phelan E, Williams B. A study of the diagnostic accuracy of the PHQ-9 in primary care elderly. *BMC Fam Pract* 2010; 11:63 www.biomedcentral.com/1471-2296/11/63/abstract

12. Kroenke K, Spitzer RL. The PHQ-9 Validity of a brief depression severity measure. *J Gen Intern Med*. 2001; 16(9):606-613 www.ncbi.nlm.nih.gov/pmc/articles/PMC1495268/?tool=pubmed

13. Cameron IM, Crawford JR. Psychometric comparison of PHQ-9 and HADS for measuring depression severity in primary care. *Br Gen Pract*. 2008; 58(546):32-36. www.ncbi.nlm.nih.gov/pmc/articles/PMC2148236/?tool=pubmed

14. Cameron IM, Lawton K. Appropriateness of antidepressant prescribing: an observational study in a Scottish primary-care setting. *Br Gen Pract* 2009; 59(566):644-649 www.ncbi.nlm.nih.gov/pmc/articles/PMC2734353/?tool=pubmed

Chapter 9 Who decides what doctors do: pharma, politicians of patients?

1. Doll R, Hill AB. Smoking and Carcinoma of the Lung. *BMJ* 1950; 2(4682):739-748 www.bmj.com/content/2/4682/739.full.pdf

2. Stead LF, Bergson G. Physician advice for smoking cessation. *Cochrane Database Syst Rev*. 2008; 16(2) www.thecochranelibrary.com/userfiles/ccoch/file/World%20No%20Tobacco%20Day/CD000165.pdf

3. Doll R, Peto R. Mortality in relation to smoking: 50 years' observations on male British Doctors. *BMJ* 2004; 328(7455) www.bmj.com/content/328/7455/1519.full

4. House of Commons Health Committee. The influence of the pharmaceutical industry. Fourth Report of Session 2004-2005 www.publications.parliament.uk/pa/cm200405/cmselect/cmhealth/42/42.pdf

5. Gagnon M-A, Lexchin J. The cost of pushing pills: a new estimate of pharmaceutical promotion expenditures in the United States. *PLoS Medicine* 2008; 5(1) www.plosmedicine.org/article/info:doi/10.1371/journal.pmed.0050001

6. IMS. New Models, New Metrics – website accessed February 2012 www.imshealth.com

7. Matyas V. Protecting the identity of doctors in drug prescription analysis. *Health Informatics Journal* 1998, 4(3):205-209 jhi.sagepub.com/content/4/3-4/205

8. Panush RS. Why I no longer accept pens (or other "gifts" from Industry (and why you shouldn't either). *J Rheumatol* 2003;31:8 www.jrheum.com/subscribers/04/08/tables/PDF/2004-38.aug.pdf

9. Fischer MA, Keough ME. Prescribers and pharmaceutical representatives: why are

we still meeting? *J Gen Intern Med.* 2009; 24(7):795-801 www.ncbi.nlm.nih.gov/pmc/articles/PMC2695530/?tool=pubmed

10. Spilker B. The benefits and risks of a pack of M&Ms, *Health Affairs* 2002 content. healthaffairs.org/content/21/2/243.full

11. Caudill TS, Johnson MS. Physicians, pharmaceutical sales representatives, and the cost of prescribing. *Arch Fam Med.* 1996; 5:201-206 archfami.ama-assn.org/cgi/reprint/5/4/201

12. Wazana A. Physicians and the pharmaceutical industry: is a gift ever just a gift? *JAMA* 2000; 283(3):373-380 jama.ama-assn.org/content/283/3/373.long

13. Irving R. GPs accused of 'Luddism' over drugs. *The Sunday Times*, June 06 2005

14. LaMattina JL. *Drug Truths: Dispelling the Myths about Pharma R&D* Wiley, 2009

15. Moreno C, Laje G. National trends in the outpatient diagnosis and treatment of bipolar disorder in youth. *Arch Gen Psychiatry* 2007; 64(9):1032-1039 archpsyc.ama-assn.org/cgi/content/abstract/64/9/1032

16. Zimmerman M, Ruggero CJ. Is bipolar disorder overdiagnosed? *J Clin Psychiatry.* 2008; 69(6):935-940 www.ncbi.nlm.nih.gov/pubmed/18466044

17. Review of the week: when truth lies buried. *BMJ* 2010; 340 www.bmj.com/content/340/bmj.c604.extract

18. Pharmaceutical giant AstraZeneca to pay $520 million for off-label drug marketing. The United States Department of Justice, April 2010 www.justice.gov/opa/pr/2010/April/10-civ-487.html

19. AstraZeneca in $198m claim payout. *BBC News Business*, August 2010 www.bbc.co.uk/news/business-10912302

20. Spielmans CI, Parry PI. From evidence-based medicine to marketing-based medicine: evidence from internal industry documents. *Bioethical Inquiry* December 2009 i.bnet.com/blogs/spielmans-parry-ebm-to-mbm-jbioethicinqu-2010.pdf

21. Bombardier C, Laine L. Comparison of upper gastrointestinal toxicity of rofecoxib and naproxen in patients with rheumatoid arthritis. *N Engl J Med* 2000; 343:1520-1528 www.nejm.org/doi/full/10.1056/NEJM200011233432103

22. Topol EJ. Failing the Public Health – Rofecoxib, Merck and the FDA. *N Engl J Med* 2004; 351:1707-1709. www.nejm.org/doi/full/10.1056/NEJMp048286

23. Curfman GD, Morrissey S. Expression of Concern: Bombardier et al., 'Comparison of Upper Gastrointestinal Toxicity of Rofecoxib and Naproxen in patients with Rheumatoid Arthritis". *N Engl J Med* 2000; 343:1520-1528. www.nejm.org/doi/full/10.1056/NEJMe058314

24. Merck News Release, April 28th, 2000 'Merck Reconfirms Favourable Cardiovascular Safety of Vioxx' dida.library.ucsf.edu/pdf/oxx17k10

25. Bresalier RS, Sandler RS. Cardiovascular events associated with Rofecoxib in a colorectal adenoma chemoprevention trial. *N Engl J Med* 2005; 352:1092-1102. www.nejm.org/doi/full/10.1056/NEJMoa050493

26. Merck Press Release. Merck announces voluntary worldwide withdrawal of VIOXX. www.merck.com/newsroom/vioxx/pdf/vioxx_press_release_final.pdf

27. Jüni P, Nartey L. Risk of cardiovascular events and rofecoxib: cumulative meta-analysis. *Lancet* 2004; 364(9450):2021-2029 www.thelancet.com/journals/lancet/article/PIIS0140-6736(04)17514-4/fulltext

28. Vioxx, the implosion of Merck, and the aftershocks at the FDA. *Lancet* 2004 364;9450:1995-1996 www.thelancet.com/journals/lancet/article/PIIS0140-6736(04)17523-5/fulltext

29. Newman M. The Rules of Retraction, *BMJ* 2010; 341: c6985 www.bmj.com/

content/341/bmj.c6985

30. Aursnes I, Tvete IF. Suicide attempts in clinical trials with paroxetine randomised against placebo. *BMC Med* 2005; 3: 14. 2005 www.ncbi.nlm.nih.gov/pmc/articles/PMC1198229/

31. FDA proposes new warnings about suicidal thinking, behaviour in young adults who take antidepressant medications. *US Food and Drug administration*, May 2007 www.fda.gov/NewsEvents/Newsroom/PressAnnouncements/2007/ucm108905.htm

32. Major pharmaceutical firm concealed drug information: GlaxoSmithKline misled doctors about the safety of drug used to treat depression in children. Media Centre 2004. www.ag.ny.gov/media_center/2004/jun/jun2b_04.html

33. Chalmers I. Government regulation is needed to prevent biased under-reporting of clinical trials. *BMJ* 2004; 329:462 www.bmj.com/content/329/7463/462.2.full

34. Clark B, *The Fight of my Life*. Hodder, 2007

35. Instant cure-all: cancer drug must be fast-tracked. *The Guardian* May 2005 www.guardian.co.uk/news/2005/may/22/leaders.comment

36. ABC News, The Top 10 Medical Advances of the Decade. 17/12/09 abcnews.go.com/Health/Decade/genome-hormones-top-10-medical-advances-decade/story?id=9356853&page=5

37. Tuma RS. Trastuzumab trials steal show at ASCO meeting. *J Natl Cancer Inst* 2005; 97(12):870-871 jnci.oxfordjournals.org/content/97/12/870.full

38. ASCO. Advances in Monoclonal antibody therapy for breast cancer www.asco.org/ascov2/MultiMedia/Virtual+Meeting?&vmview=vm_session_presentations_view&confID=34&sessionID=1708

39. Romond EH, Perez EA. Trastuzumab plus adjuvant chemotherapy for operable HER2-positive breast cancer. *N Engl J Med* 2005; 353:1673-1684 www.nejm.org/doi/full/10.1056/NEJMoa052122

40. Hortobagyi GN. Trastuzumab in the treatment of Breast cancer. *N Engl J Med* 2005; 353:1734-1736 www.nejm.org/doi/full/10.1056/NEJMe058196

41. Herceptin trastuzumab. Adjuvant Breast cancer treatment clinical study results www.herceptin.com/hcp/treatment/adjuvant/studies.html

42. Guarneri V, Lenihan DJ. Long-term cardiac tolerability of trastuzumab in metastatic breast cancer: the MD Anderson Cancer Centre experience. *J Clin Oncol* 2006; 24(25):4107-4115 jco.ascopubs.org/content/24/25/4107.long

43. Riccart-Gebhart MJ, Procter M. Trastuzumab after Adjuvant chemotherapy in HER2-Positive Breast Cancer. *N Engl J Med* 2005;353:1659-1672 www.nejm.org/doi/full/10.1056/NEJMoa052306

44. Breastcancer.org Corporate Partners www.breastcancer.org/about_us/supporters/corp_sponsors.jsp

45. Romond EH, Edith MD. Trastuzumab plus adjuvant chemotherapy for Operable HER2-Positive breast cancer. *N Engl J Med* 2005; 353:1673-1684

46. Dolan A. 'My mum has breast cancer, please save her'. *The Daily Mail*, March 2006 www.dailymail.co.uk/health/article-379338/My-mum-breast-cancer-save-her.html

47. McCartney M. Are we educating women to be afraid? *Cancerworld* www.cancerworld.org/Articles/Issues_32/Best_Cancer_Reporter_Award/Are_we_educating_women_to_be_afraid%3F%

Chapter 10 Charities and favourite diseases

1. New survey reveals severity of stroke still widely underestimated. The Stroke Association, October 2004 www.stroke.org.uk/media_centre/press_releases/new_

survey.html

2. Too many elderly 'left in pain'. *BBC News* Online October 2006 news.bbc.co.uk/1/hi/health/6065754.stm

3. Equity and excellence: liberating the NHS. Terrence Higgins Trust October 2010 www.tht.org.uk/binarylibrary/policy/commissioning-white-paper-response.pdf

4. Why awareness matters. Target Ovarian Cancer www.targetovariancancer.org.uk/page.asp?section=97&sectionTitle=Raising+awareness+of+ovarian+cancer+symptoms

5. Written evidence from Arrhythmia Alliance (COM 114). www.parliament.uk October 2010 www.publications.parliament.uk/pa/cm201011/cmselect/cmhealth/513/513vw108.htm

6. Breast cancer campaigning lauded for Herceptin case. Brand Republic, March 2006 www.brandrepublic.com/news/544082/Breast-Cancer-Campaign-lauded-Herceptin-case/?DCMP=ILC-SEARCH

7. Keiden J. Sucked into the Herceptin maelstrom. *BMJ* 2007; 334:18 www.bmj.com/content/334/7583/18?variant=full

8. Breast Cancer Campaign, May 2006 breastcancercampaign.org/

9. Breast Cancer Network Australia Campaigns www.bcna.org.au/about-bcna/advocacy/campaigns

10. Herceptin and early breast cancer: a moment for caution. *Lancet* 2005; 366(9498):1673 www.thelancet.com/journals/lancet/article/PIIS0140-6736(05)67670-2/fulltext

11. Aukland Women's Health Council, Herceptin www.womenshealthcouncil.org.nz/Features/Hot+Topics/Herceptin.html

12. British Skin Foundation. About the BSF. www.britishskinfoundation.org.uk/AboutUs.aspx

13. Dr. Nick Lowe Dermatologist. Skin Solutions. www.drnicklowe.com/

14. Heart UK: The Cholesterol Charity www.heartuk.org.uk/index.php?/about_us/heart_uk_partners1/

15. IBS Network. Our partners. www.theibsnetwork.org/ourpartners.asp

16. Breast Cancer Breakthrough. Partner your brand with us. www.breakthrough.org.uk/corporate_partners/work_with_us/

17. Breast Cancer Breakthrough. Financial Support 2008/09. www.breakthrough.org.uk/corporate_partners/work_with_pharmaceutical_companies/financial_support_09.html

18. Trustee's report and financial statements. Parkinson's Disease Society of the United Kingdom (Parkinson's UK), December 2009 www.parkinsons.org.uk/docs/annualreport2009.pdf

19. GlaxoSmithKline, Responsibility, Commitment to transparency. Patient group funding. Accessed February 2012 www.gsk.com/responsibility/patient-groups/uk-po-asthma-uk.htm

20. Asthma UK, Corporate Gold and Silver. Accessed February 2012 www.asthma.org.uk/corporate_partners/corporate_gold_and_s.html

21. www.diabetes.org.uk/Diabetes-UK-Professional-Conference/Registration/Information-on-funding

22. GSK. Patient group funding www.gsk.com/responsibility/patient-groups/uk-po-diabetes-uk.htm

23. Letter to *The Times*, 24/2/10 Patient wellbeing at risk from substituted generic medicines. http://www.thetimes.co.uk/tto/opinion/letters/article2072558.ece

24. McCartney M. Generic drugs: protest group was not quite what it seemed. *BMJ* 2010; 340:c1514 www.bmj.com/content/340/bmj.c1514.full

25. Ball DE, Tisocki K. Advertising and disclosure of funding on patient organisation websites: a cross-sectional survey. *BMC Public Health* 2006; 6:201 www.ncbi.nlm.nih. gov/pmc/articles/PMC1557495/

26. Vermeulen M, Bouma J. The influence of the pharmaceutical industry in patient organisations. *Ned Tijdschr Geneeskd* 2007; 151(44):2432-2434 www.ncbi.nlm.nih.gov/pubmed/18064861

27. Jones K. In whose interest? Relationships between health consumer groups and the pharmaceutical industry in the UK. *Sociol Health Illn* 2008; 30(6):929-943 www.ncbi. nlm.nih.gov/pubmed/18761512

28. CoppaFeel! coppafeel.org/page/boobcheck

29. Male Cancer Awareness Campaign www.malecancer.org/abouts

30. Who's in the House? Male Cancer Awareness Campaign, March 2010 www. malecancer.org/featured_articles/item/14

31. Information on Testicular Cancer, Orchid: Fighting Male Cancer Leaflets. www. orchid-cancer.org.uk/453/Know-Your-Balls-Check-em-Out

32. Macmillan Cancer Information www.macmillan.org.uk/Cancerinformation/ Cancertypes/Testes/Symptomsdiagnosis/Checkum.aspx

33. McCartney, M. How useful are lifetime risks of disease? *BMJ* 2011; 342 doi: 10.1136/ bmj.d1046 www.bmj.com/content/342/bmj.d1046

34. Phillips KA, Glendon G. Putting the risk of breast cancer in perspective. *N Engl J Med* 1999; 340(2): 141-144 www.nejm.org/doi/full/10.1056/NEJM199901143400211

35. Smith BL, Gadd MA. Perception of breast cancer risk among women in breast centre and primary care setting: correlation with age and family history of breast cancer. *Surgery* 1996; 120(2): 297-303 www.surgjournal.com/article/S0039-6060(96)80301-1/ abstract

36. Moser K, Patnick J, Beral V. Do women know that the risk of breast cancer increases with age? *Brit J Gen Pract*, 2007, 57(538) 404-406 www.ncbi.nlm.nih.gov/pmc/articles/ PMC2047017/?tool=pubmed

37. Cummings KM, Lampone D. What young men know about testicular cancer. *Prev Med.* 1983; 12(2):326-330 www.ncbi.nlm.nih.gov/pubmed/6878194

38. Moore RA, Topping A. Young men's knowledge of testicular cancer and testicular self-examination: a lost opportunity? *Eur J Cancer Care* (Engl) 1999; 8(3): 137-142 onlinelibrary.wiley.com/doi/10.1046/j.1365-2354.1999.00151.x/abstract

39. Cancer Research UK. Testicular Cancer statistics. info.cancerresearchuk.org/ cancerstats/types/testis/

40. Thomas DB, Gao DL. Randomized trial of breast self-examination in Shanghai: Final results. *J Natl Cancer Inst* 2002; 94(19):1445-1457 jnci.oxfordjournals.org/ content/94/19/1445.long

41. Cancer Research UK cancer statistics info.cancerresearchuk.org/cancerstats/types/ testis/mortality/

42. Office for National Statistical Bulletin, Suicide Rates in the United Kingdom, 2000-2009 27/1/11 http://www.ons.gov.uk/ons/rel/subnational-health4/suicides-in-the-united-kingdom/2010/index.html

43. World report chapter 1. Who Int. www.who.int/violence_injury_prevention/ publications/road_traffic/world_report/chapter1.pdf

44. Rachel Stevens 'gets fruity' for Everyman. Everyman, June 2005 everyman-campaign. org/News/Press_Archive/2005/13480.shtml

45. Thornhill JA, Fennelly JJ. Patients' delay in the presentation of testis cancer in Ireland. *Br J Urol.* 1987; 59(5):447-451 onlinelibrary.wiley.com/doi/10.1111/j.1464-410X.1987.

tb04844.x/abstract

46. Vasudev NS, Joffe JK. Delay in the diagnosis of testicular tumours – changes over the past 18 years. *Br Gen Pract*. 2004; 54(505):595-597 www.ingentaconnect.com/content/rcgp/bjgp/2004/00000054/00000505/art00008

47. Khadra A, Oakeshott P. Pilot study of testicular cancer awareness and testicular self-examination in men attending two South London general practices. *Fam Pract*. 202; 19(3): 294-296 fampra.oxfordjournals.org/content/19/3/294.full

48. At-risk men 'unaware' of cancer threat. *BBC News*, June 1999 news.bbc.co.uk/1/hi/health/359443.stm

49. Gascoigne P, Mason MD. Factors affecting presentation and delay in patients with testicular cancer: results of a qualitative study. *Psychooncology* 1999; 8(2):144-154 onlinelibrary.wiley.com/doi/10.1002/(SICI)1099-1611(199903/04)8:2%3C144::AID-PON349%3E3.0.CO;2-P/abstract

50. Breakthrough breast cancer. Breast awareness. www.breakthrough.org.uk/breast_cancer/breast_awareness/

51. The Prostate Cancer Charity. Prostate and prostate cancer FAQs. www.prostate-cancer.org.uk/information/faq

52. Neate J. Let men make informed choices on prostate cancer screening. *The Guardian*, December 2010 www.guardian.co.uk/commentisfree/2010/dec/08/prostate-screening-campaign

53. Prostate Screening Trust www.prostatescreeningtrust.co.uk/

54. Kao T-C, Cruess DF. Multicentre patient self-reporting questionnaire on impotence, incontinence and stricture after radical prostatectomy. *J Urolology* 200; 163(3):858-864. www.jurology.com/article/S0022-5347(05)67819-6/abstract

55. Volk RJ, Hawley ST. Trials of decision aids for prostate cancer screening: a systematic review. *Am J Prev Med* 2007; 33(5):428-434 www.ajpmonline.org/article/S0749-3797(07)00497-7/abstract

56. Frosch DL, Kaplan RM. The evaluation of two methods to facilitate shared decision making for men considering the prostate-specific antigen test. *J Gen Intern Med* 2001; 16(6):391-398 www.ncbi.nlm.nih.gov/pmc/articles/PMC1495230/

57. For the man in your life . . . ignorance isn't bliss: a woman's guide to the prostate. Prostate UK 2004

Chapter 11 The problem with PR

1. Advert in the *Guardian* newspaper, 2006 www.margaretmccartney.com/blog/?attachment_id=1256&cpage=1#comment-3381

2. British Heart Foundation. Job vacancy https://jobs.bhf.org.uk/admin/Files/Public/Vacancies/152/User26/Celebrity%20Liaison%20&%20Media%20Officer%20JD%202010.pdf

3. Hope hits the headlines. British Heart Foundation, February 2011 www.bhf.org.uk/default.aspx?page=12830

4. Macrae F. Pill that can trick your heart into fixing itself. *The Mail Online*. February 2011 www.dailymail.co.uk/health/article-1352257/Pill-allows-damaged-hearts-repair-available-seven-years.htm

5. D'Souza R. British Scientists create miracle pill to mend broken hearts. *Manufacturing Digital*, 2011. www.manufacturingdigital.com/sectors/british-scientists-create-miracle-pill-mend-broken-hearts

6. Alleyne R. Recovering from a heart attack could soon be as simple as recovering from a broken leg. *The Telegraph* February 2011 www.telegraph.co.uk/health/

healthnews/8293320/Recovering-from-a-heart-attack-could-soon-be-as-simple-as-recovering-f

7. British Heart Foundation. The Science. www.bhf.org.uk/research/mending-broken-hearts-appeal/the-science.aspx

8. Whitcroft I. How a prostate test taught Darth Vader he's not so invincible after all. *Mail Online*, December 2009 www.dailymail.co.uk/health/article-1239014/How-prostate-test-taught-Darth-Vader-hes-invincible-all.html

9. Estee Lauder. Pink Ribbon Collection. www.esteelauder.com.au/cms/about/breast_cancer_awareness_index.tmpl

10. McCartney M. One in four women? *FT Health and Science blog*, October 2009 blogs.ft.com/healthblog/2009/10/26/one-in-four-women/#axzz1i7p3cJx4

11. Annual report and audited financial statements. Hyperlipidaemia education & atherosclerosis research trust UK (Heart UK), February 2010 www.heartuk.org.uk/images/uploads/aboutuspdfs/Annual_Report_10.pdf

12. Heart UK. Product Approval www.heartuk.org.uk/index.php?/about_us/product_approval/

13. Landmark Study: Pravastatin rapidly reduces risk of heart attacks and saves lives of people with high cholesterol and no previous heart attack. Press Release 15th November 1995 www.gla.ac.uk/departments/vascularbiochemistry/research/woscops/resultsandconclusions/

14. Shepherd J, Cobbe SM. Prevention of Coronary Heart Disease with Pravastatin in Men with Hypercholesterolemia *N Eng J Med* 1995; 333:1301-1308 www.nejm.org/doi/full/10.1056/NEJM199511163332001

15. Skolbekken J-A. Communicating the risk reduction achieved by cholesterol reducing drugs. *BMJ* 1998; 316:1956 www.bmj.com/content/316/7149/1956.full

16. Wald N, Law MR. A strategy to reduce cardiovascular disease by more than 80%. *BMJ* 2003; 326:1419 www.bmj.com/content/326/7404/1419.full

17. Smith R. The most important BMJ for 50 years? *BMJ* 2003: 326 www.bmj.com/content/326/7404/0.7.full

18. Hippisley-Cox J, Coupland C. Unintended effects of statins in men and women in England and Wales: population based cohort study using the QResearch database. *BMJ* 2010; 340:c2197 www.bmj.com/content/340/bmj.c2197.abstract

19. Mayer B, Baggio C. Gastroprotective constituents of Salvua officinalis L. *Fitoterapia* 2009; 80(7): 421-426 www.ncbi.nlm.nih.gov/pubmed/19481590

20. Is sage the new superfood? Elsevier 'Flash' press release, 6/10/09

21. Boutron I, Dutton S. Reporting and interpretation of randomized controlled trials with statistically nonsignificant results for primary outcomes. *JAMA* 2010; 303(2):2058-2064 jama.ama-assn.org/content/303/20/2058.short

22. Berwanger O, Ribeiro RA. The quality of reporting of trial abstracts is suboptimal: survey of major general medical journals. *J Clin Epidemiol* 2009; 62(4):387-392 www.jclinepi.com/article/S0895-4356(08)00223-0/abstract

23. Select Committee on science and technology (third report). Chapter 7: Science and the media. Parliament.uk www.publications.parliament.uk/pa/ld199900/ldselect/ldsctech/38/3810.htm

24. Woloshin S. Schwartz LM. Press releases by academic medical centres: Not so academic? www.annals.org/content/150/9/613.full.pdf+html

25. Moynihan R, Bero L. Coverage by the news media of the benefits and risks of medications. *N Engl J Med* 2000; 342:1645-1650 www.nejm.org/doi/full/10.1056/NEJM200006013422206

26. Find your me spot www.findyourmespot.com/what.htm
27. Incredibull: Find your me spot campaign incredibull3.drupalgardens.com/casestudies/bayer-find-your-me-spot
28. Sleep Well, Live Well www.sleepwelllivewell.co.uk/
29. www.sleepwelllivewell.co.uk/PATIENT%20LEAFLET.pdf
30. Incredibull: Live Well, Sleep well incredibull3.drupalgardens.com/casestudies/lundbeck
31. Buscemi N, Vandermeer B. The efficacy and safety of exogenous melatonin for primary sleep disorders. *J Gen Intern Med* 2005; 20(12):1151-1158 www.ncbi.nlm.nih.gov/pmc/articles/PMC1490287/?tool=pubmed
32. Buscemi N, Vandermeer B. Efficacy and safety of exogenous melatonin for secondary sleep disorders and sleep disorders accompanying sleep restriction: meta-analysis. *BMJ* 2006; 332:385 www.bmj.com/content/332/7538/385?view=long&pmid=16473858
33. Press Release. MMYM Launches New Chlamydia Screening Programme in Shropshire. 21/10/10 www.pressbox.co.uk/detailed/Health/MMYM_Launches_New_Chlamydia_Screening_Programme_in_Shropshire_562786.html
34. The Comptroller and Auditor General. Young people's sexual health: the National chlamydia screening programme. National Audit Office, November 2009 www.nao.org.uk/publications/0809/young_peoples_sexual_health.aspx
35. Low N, Bender N. Effectiveness of chlamydia screening: systematic review. *Int J Epidemiol* 2009; 38(2):435-448 ije.oxfordjournals.org/content/38/2/435.abstract
36. O'Reilly E. Mpad wins Chlamydia testing brief. PR Week, 20 October 2008 www.prweek.com/uk/news/854935/Mpad-wins-chlamydia-testing-brief/
37. www.sandyford.org/media/113992/sexual%20and%20reproductive%20health%20primary%20care%20guidelines.pdf
38. Akande V, Turner C. Impact of Chlamydia Trachomatis in the reproductive setting: British Fertility Society guideline for practice. *Hum Fertil* (CamB). 2010; 13(3):115-125 ukpmc.ac.uk/articles/PMC3069694
30. Frisky not risky chlamydia screening (case study). PMLive Intelligence online, October 2010 www.pmlive.com/pharma_news/frisky_not_risky_223981

Chapter 12 Professionals in pay

1. Press release HARDSPR 2/8/10 stored at www.margaretmccartney.com/blog/?p=1257
2. Markey CN, Markey PM. A correlational and experimental examination of reality television viewing and interest in cosmetic surgery. *Body Image* 2010; 7(2):165-171 www.ncbi.nlm.nih.gov/pubmed/20089464
3. Haas CF, Champion A, Secor D. Motivating factors for seeking cosmetic surgery: a synthesis of the literature. *Past Surg Nurs.* 2008; 28(4):177-182 journals.lww.com/psnjournalonline/Abstract/2008/10000/Motivating_Factors_for_Seeking_Cosmetic_Surgery__A.6.aspx
4. Calogero RM, Park LE. Predicting excessive body image concerns among British university students: the unique role of appearance-based rejection sensitivity. *Body Image* 2010; 7(1): 78-81 www.sciencedirect.com/science/article/pii/S1740144509000977
5. Veale D. Body dysmorphic disorder. *Postgrad Med J* 2004; 80:67-71 pmj.bmj.com/content/80/940/67.full
6. Mya cosmetic vaginal surgery www.mya.co.uk/cosmetic-surgery/vaginal-surgery.php
7. Castle DJ, Honigman RJ. Does cosmetic surgery improve psychosocial wellbeing? *MJA* 2002; 176(12): 601-604 www.mja.com.au/public/issues/176_12_170602/cas10571_

fm.html

8. Bruck JC, Kleinschmidt A. Increased self-confidence and decreased sexual discomfort after subpectoral mammoplasty. *Handchir Mikrochir Plast Chir*. 2001; 43(2):112-118 www.ncbi.nlm.nih.gov/pubmed/21132627

9. More magazine Stored at www.margaretmccartney.com/blog/?p=1265

10. Hirsch L. Five secrets to leveraging maximum buying power with your media project. *Facial Plastic Surgery Clinics of North America* 2010; 18(4): 525-531 www.facialplastic. theclinics.com/article/S1064-7406(10)00092-1/abstract

11. How is general practice funded? NHS History, October 2008 www.nhshistory.com/ gppay.pdf

12. Quality and outcomes framework guidance for GMS contract 2011-12. *BMA*, April 2011 www.nhsemployers.org/Aboutus/Publications/Documents/QOF_guidance_ GMS_contract_2011_12.pdf

13. Quality and outcomes framework guidance for GMS contract 2009/2010: delivering investment in general practice. BMA & NHS Employers, March 2009 www.bma.org. uk/images/qof0309_tcm41-184025.pdf

14. Patient Health Questionnaire (PHQ) Screeners. Screener Overview. www. phqscreeners.com/overview.aspx

15. The PHQ-9 works well as a screening but not a diagnostic instrument for depressive disorder. *Evidence Based Mental Health* 2010; 13:96 ebmh.bmj.com/content/13/3/96. extract

16. Baker D, Middleton E. Cervical screening and health inequality in England in the 1990s. *J Epidemiol Commun H* 203; 57:419-423 jech.bmj.com/content/57/6/417. abstract

Chapter 13 Political patients

1. Hart JT. The inverse care law. *Lancet*. 1971 Feb 27; 1(7696):405-12. www.thelancet. com/journals/lancet/article/PIIS0140-6736(71)92410-X/abstract

2. Accessing therapy. NHS choices. www.nhs.uk/Livewell/counselling/Pages/ Accesstotherapy.aspx

3. Physiotherapy – Accessing physiotherapy. NHS Choices. www.nhs.uk/Conditions/ Physiotherapy/Pages/Accessing-physiotherapy.aspx

4. Brown JSL, Boardman J. Can a self-referral system help improve access to psychological treatments? *Brit J Gen Pract* 2010; 60(574):365-371 www.ncbi.nlm.nih. gov/pmc/articles/PMC2858533/?tool=pubmed

5. Clark DM, Layard R. Improving access to psychological therapy: initial evaluation of two UK demonstration sites. *Behav Res Ther* 2009; 47(11): 910-920 www.sciencedirect. com/science/article/pii/S0005796709001703

6. Bowers L. Community psychiatric nurse caseloads and the 'worried well': misspent time vital work? J Adv Nurs. 1997; 26(5):930-936 onlinelibrary.wiley.com/doi/10.1046/ j.1365-2648.1997.00436.x/abstract

7. St John-Smith P, McQueen D. The trouble with NHS psychiatry in England. Psychiatric Bulletin 2009; 33:219-225 pb.rcpsych.org/content/33/6/219

8. Green B. The decline of NHS inpatient psychiatry in England. Priory.com, March 2009 priory.com/psychiatry/Decline_NHS_Inpatient_Psychiatry.htm

9. The Royal College of Psychiatrists. In-patient services. www.rcpsych.ac.uk/campaigns/ fairdeal/whatisfairdeal/in-patientservices.aspx

10. New Roles for psychiatrists. National Working Group on New Roles for Psychiatrists February 2004. www.dh.gov.uk/en/Publicationsandstatistics/Publications/

PublicationsPolicyAndGuidance/DH_4073490

11. Pidd H. NHS Direct to be replaced by cut-price health advice service *The Guardian*, 27.08.2010 www.guardian.co.uk/politics/2010/aug/27/nhs-direct-health-phone-service

12. Self Care Campaign. About us. Accessed February 2011. www.selfcarecampaign.org/about-us

13. The Proprietary Association of Great Britain. Market figures www.pagb.co.uk/media/facts.html

14. Making the case for the self-care of minor elements. PAGB, August 2009 www.pagb.co.uk/publications/pdfs/Minorailmentsresearch09.pdf

15. Davies P. Darzi centres: an expensive luxury the UK can no longer afford? *BMJ* 2010; 341 www.bmj.com/content/341/bmj.c6287?papetoc=

16. Iacobucci G. GP-led health centres 'dominated by nurses and salaried doctors'. *Pulse*, Feb 2009 www.pulsetoday.co.uk/newsarticle-content/-/article_display_list/10997436/gp-led-health-centres-dominated-by-nurses-and-salaried-doctors

17. Lord Darzi's white elephant legacy. *Pulse*, 4th Nov 2009. www.pulsetoday.co.uk/main-content/-/article_display_list/11017006/lord-darzi-s-white-elephant-legacy

18. Irvine M-L. Darzi centres are an expensive instant minor illness service *BMJ*, 2010 www.bmj.com/rapid-response/2011/11/03/darzi-centres-are-expensive-instant-minor-illness-service

19. Iacobucci G. Darzi centre dwarfs GMS cash. Pulse, July 2009 www.pulsetoday.co.uk/newsarticle-content/-/article_display_list/11008998/darzi-centre-funding-dwarfs-gms-cash

20. NHS Choose and book. Clinical responsibilities when delegating actions in NHS choose and book. www.chooseandbook.nhs.uk/staff/communications/fact/clinicalrespons.pdf

21. Quinn I. Radical new gateways reject one in eight GP referrals. *Pulse*, February 2011 www.pulsetoday.co.uk/newsarticle-content/-/article_display_list/11053620/radical-new-gateways-reject-one-in-eight-gp

22. Gateways using nurses to screen GP referrals. *Pulse*, August 2011 www.pulsetoday.co.uk/main-content/-/article_display_list/12511567/gateways-using-nurses-to-screen-gp-refe

23. Davies M, Elwyn G. Referral management centres: promising innovations or Trojan Horses? *BMJ*, 2006; 332:844 www.bmj.com/content/332/7545/844?variant=full

24. Referral management centres fail to deliver savings, according to new research from The King's fund. The King's Fund, August 2010 www.kingsfund.org.uk/press/press_releases/referral_management.html

25. Potter S, Govindarajulu S. Referral patterns, cancer diagnoses, and waiting times after introduction of two week wait rule for breast cancer: prospective cohort study. *BMJ* 2007; 335:288 www.bmj.com/content/early/2006/12/31/bmj.39258.688553.55.full

26. GPRD www.gprd.com/home/

27. Jones R, Charlton J. Alarm Symptoms and identification of non-cancer diagnoses in primary care: cohort study. *BMJ* 2009; 339 www.bmj.com/content/339/bmj.b3094.full

28. Rossing MA, Wicklund KG. Predictive value of symptoms for early detection of ovarian cancer. *JNCI* 2010; 102(4):222-229 jnci.oxfordjournals.org/content/102/4/222.abstract

29. Bankhead CR, Collins C. Identifying symptoms of ovarian cancer: a qualitative and quantitative study. *BJOG* 2008; 115(8):1008-1014 www.ncbi.nlm.nih.gov/pmc/articles/PMC2607526/?tool=pubmed

30. Hamilton W, Lancashire R. The risk of colorectal cancer with symptoms at different ages and between the sexes: a case-control study. *BMC Medicine* 2009; 7:17 www.biomedcentral.com/1741-7015/7/17

31. Jones R. Is the two week rule for cancer referrals working? BMJ 2001; 322:1555 www.bmj.com/content/322/7302/1555.full

32. Thorne K, Hutchings HA. The two-week rule for NHS Gastrointestinal Cancer referrals: A systematic review of diagnostic effectiveness. The Open Colorectal Cancer Journal 2009; 2:27-33 www.biomedcentral.com/1472-6963/6/43

33. Lewis NR. Jeune IL. Under utilisation of the 2-week wait initiative for lung cancer by primary care and its effect on the urgent referral pathway. British Journal of Cancer 2005; 93:905-908. www.ncbi.nlm.nih.gov/pmc/articles/PMC2361660/

34. Potter S, Govindarajulu S. Referral patterns, cancer diagnoses, and waiting times after introduction of two week wait rule for breast cancer: prospective cohort study. BMJ 2007; 335:288 www.bmj.com/content/335/7614/288.abstract

35. Hanna SJ, Muneer A. The 2-week wait for suspected cancer: a time for rethink? International Journal of Clinical Practice 2005; 59(11):1334-1339 onlinelibrary.wiley.com/doi/10.1111/j.1368-5031.2005.00687.x/full

Chapter 14 What sort of patient?

1. www.nhsdirect.nhs.uk/News/PressReleases/~/media/Files/2007PressReleases/PR_181007_NHSDLaunchesNewPatientSupportProgramme.ashx

2. Mansell P. The patient paradox. *Pharma Times* Oct 2010 www.pharmatimes.com/documents/2010/October/the%20patient%20paradox.pdf

3. Department of Health. Improving Chronic Disease Management. www.dh.gov.uk/prod_consum_dh/groups/dh_digitalassets/@dh/@en/documents/digitalasset/dh_4075213.pdf

4. National Primary Care Research & Development Centre www.medicine.manchester.ac.uk/primarycare/npcrdc-archive/archive/

5. Kennedy A, Gately C. Assessing the Process of embedding EPP in the NHS preliminary survey of PCT Pilot sites. National Primary Care Research and Development Centre, January 2004. www.medicine.manchester.ac.uk/primarycare/npcrdc-archive/Publications/EPP%20Report%202004.pdf

6. Richardson G, Kennedy A. Cost effectiveness of Expert Patients Programme (EPP) for patients with chronic conditions. *J Epidemiol Commun H* 2008; 62:361-367 jech.bmj.com/content/62/4/361.abstract

7. Phillips C. What is a QALY? What is...? Series, April 2009 www.medicine.ox.ac.uk/bandolier/painres/download/whatis/QALY.pdf

8. Foster G, Taylor SJC. Self-management education programmes by lay leaders for people with chronic conditions. *The Cochrane Library*, Jan 2009 onlinelibrary.wiley.com/doi/10.1002/14651858.CD005108.pub2/pdf/standard

9. Rogers A, Gately C. Are some more equal than others? Social comparison in self-management skills training for long-term conditions. *Chronic Illness* 2009; 5(4):305-317 chi.sagepub.com/content/5/4/305.abstract

10. National Primary Care Research and Development Centre. Expert Patients Programme (EPP): national evaluation. NRCRDC archive site, December 2010. www.medicine.manchester.ac.uk/primarycare/npcrdc-archive/archive/ProjectDetail.cfm/ID/117.htm

11. Expert Patients Programme. About us www.expertpatients.co.uk/about-us/facts-and-figures

12. General Medical Council. Duties of a doctor www.gmc-uk.org/guidance/good_ medical_practice/duties_of_a_doctor.asp

13. Lansley A. Equity and excellence: Liberating the NHS. Press release, July 2010. www. dh.gov.uk/en/MediaCentre/Pressreleases/DH_117360

14. Office for National Statistics. News release: 9.2 million UK adults have never used the internet. August 2010 http://www.ons.gov.uk/ons/rel/rdit2/internet-access---households-and-individuals/2010/index.html

15. Hoffman, J. Awash with information, patients face a lonely, uncertain road. *New York Times*, August 2005 www.nytimes.com/2005/08/14/health/14patient.html?pagewanted=all

16. General Medical Council. Good Medical Practice: Doctor patient partnership. www.gmc-uk.org/guidance/good_medical_practice/relationships_with_patients_partnership.asp

17. Department of Health. Liberating the NHS: Greater choice and control. 18/10/10 consultations.dh.gov.uk/choice/choice

18. Parlimentary questions, Ben Bradshaw, 24/4/98 www.publications.parliament.uk/pa/cm200708/cmhansrd/cm080424/text/80424w0002.htm

19. Gould M. Claims that NHS choose and book system puts choice before quality. *The Guardian*, March 2010 www.guardian.co.uk/society/2010/mar/24/hospital-appointments-system-choose-book

20. Nowottny S. Revealed: Choose and Book to cost taxpayers £210m. *Pulse*, October 2011. www.pulsetoday.co.uk/newsarticle-content/-/article_display_list/10950416/revealed-choose-and-book-to-cost-taxpayers-210m

21. Carvel J. Patients to rate and review their GPs on NHS website. *The Guardian* 2008 www.guardian.co.uk/society/2008/dec/30/doctors-rating-website-nhs

Chapter 15 Not more information, better information

1. NHS Evidence. UK DUETs: A resource to make uncertainties explicit and to help prioritise new research www.library.nhs.uk/DUETs/page.aspx?pagename=UNCERT

2. Johnson RT, Dickersin K. Publication bias against negative results from clinical trials. Nature Reviews Neurology 2007; 3:590-591 www.nature.com/nrneurol/journal/v3/n11/full/ncpneuro0618.html

3. Bandyopadhyay S, Bayer AJ. Age and gender bias in statin trials. *QJM* 2001; 94(3):127-132 qjmed.oxfordjournals.org/content/94/3/127.abstract

4. Murthy VK, Krumholz HM. Participation in cancer clinical trials. *JAMA* 2004; 291(22):2720-2726 jama.ama-assn.org/content/291/22/2720.abstract

5. The NNT (The Number Needed to Treat). Glucocorticoids (steroids) for Croup www.thennt.com/steroids-for-croup/

6. McMenamin M, Barry H. A survey of breast cancer awareness and knowledge in a Western population: lots of light but little illumination. *European Journal of Cancer* 2005; 41(3):393-397 www.ejcancer.info/article/S0959-8049(04)00974-8/abstract

7. Evans R, Edwards A. Reduction in uptake of PSA tests following decision aids: systematic review of current aids and their evaluations. *Patient Education and Counselling* 2005; 58(1):13-26 www.pec-journal.com/article/S0738-3991(04)00199-5/abstract

8. Smith SK, Trevena L. A decision aid to support informed choices about bowel cancer screening among adults with low education: randomised controlled trial. *BMJ* 2010; 341:c5370 www.bmj.com/content/341/bmj.c5370.full

9. Randomised controlled trial: A decision aid to support informed choice about bowel

cancer screening in people with low educational level improves knowledge but reduces screening uptake. *Evid Based Nurs* 2011; 13 ebn.bmj.com/content/early/2011/02/13/ebn1142.extract

10. Bekker HL. Decision aids and uptake of screening. *BMJ* 2010; 341:c5407 www.bmj.com/content/341/bmj.c5407

11. Arias E. United States life tables, 2006. National Vital Statistics Reports, June 2010. DHHS Publication No. (PHS) 2010-1120 www.cdc.gov/nchs/data/nvsr/nvsr58/nvsr58_21.pdf

12. Office of National Statistics. Life expectancies at birth and at age 65 in the United Kingdom. 2004-06 to 2008-10 www.ons.gov.uk/ons/dcp171778_238743.pdf

13. McNaughton-Collins M, Fowler FJ. Psychological effects of a suspicious prostate cancer screening test followed by a benign biopsy result. *Am J Med* 2004; 117(10):719-725 www.amjmed.com/article/S0002-9343(04)00542-X/abstract

14. NHS Scotland, Cervical screening put it on your list booklet, 2010 www.healthscotland.com/uploads/documents/13485-TheCervicalScreeningTest.pdf

15. Boseley S. NICE to lose powers to decide on new drugs. *The Guardian*, October 2010 www.guardian.co.uk/politics/2010/oct/29/nice-to-lose-new-drug-power

16. National Audit Office. The National programme for IT in the NHS: an update on the delivery of detailed care records systems. HC; 88:2010-2012 www.publications.parliament.uk/pa/cm201012/cmselect/cmpubacc/1070/1070.pdf

17. Pollock AM. Independent sectors treatment centres: evidence so far. *BMJ* 2008; 336:421 www.bmj.com/content/336/7641/421

18. ISTC Performance Management Analysis. Report to the Department of Health. National centre for health outcomes development, 2004 www.publications.parliament.uk/pa/cm200506/cmselect/cmhealth/934/934awe25.htm

19. Hall C. Foreign surgeons' work attacked as inferior. *The Telegraph*, February 2005 www.telegraph.co.uk/news/uknews/1483628/Foreign-surgeons-work-attacked-as-inferior.html

20. Ferris JD. Independent sector treatment centres (ISTCS): early experience from an ophthalmology perspective. *Eye* 2005; 19:1090-1098 www.nature.com/eye/journal/v19/n10/full/6702007a.html

21. Mason A, Street A. Private sector treatment centres are treating less complex patients than the NHS. *J R Soc Med* 2010; 103(8):322-331 www.ncbi.nlm.nih.gov/pmc/articles/PMC2913062/?tool=pubmed

22. Clamp JA, Baiju DSR. Do independent sector treatment centres (ISTC) Impact on specialist registrar training in primary hip and knee arthroplasty? *Ann R Coll Surg Engl.* 2008; 90(6): 492-496 www.ncbi.nlm.nih.gov/pmc/articles/PMC2647243/

23. McGauran A. It's time to rethink access to GPs within 48 hours, report says. *BMJ* 2004; 329:762 www.ncbi.nlm.nih.gov/pmc/articles/PMC521032/

24. Committee of Public Accounts. Thirty-fifth report: the refinancing of the Norfolk and Norwich PFI hospital (HC 694). Press Notice 2006; 35: Session 2005-06 www.parliament.uk/business/committees/committees-archive/committee-of-public-accounts/pac030506-pn35/

25. Limb M. PFI deals need more scrutiny after shareholders receive big windfalls. *BMJ* 2005; 330:1407 www.bmj.com/content/331/7512/343.3

26. Private Finance Initiatives during NHS austerity, Pollock AM, Price D, *BMJ* 2011; 342:d324 www.bmj.com/content/342/bmj.d324

27. Starr J. Hospital acquired infection. *BMJ* 2007; 334:708 www.bmj.com/content/334/7596/708.extract

28. NHS National Patient Safety Agency. Clean your hands www.npsa.nhs.uk/cleanyourhands/

29. Dentith M, Shelmerdine T. Organising an awareness week to target hand hygiene practice. Nursing Times 2004; 100(17):36 www.nursingtimes.net/nursing-practice-clinical-research/organising-an-awareness-week-to-target-hand-hygiene-practice/204413.article

30. Department of Health. Uniforms and workwear: an evidence base for developing local policy. September 2007 www.dh.gov.uk/prod_consum_dh/groups/dh_digitalassets/documents/digitalasset/dh_078435.pdf

31. Sears N. Yo! Middle-aged nurses make cringeworthy Ali G-style rap video to encourage cleanliness. The Daily Mail, September 2010 www.dailymail.co.uk/news/article-1308807/Ali-G-style-rap-video-NHS-staff-branded-absurd-patronising.html

32. Davies S. Fragmented management, hospital contract cleaning and infection control. Policy & Politics 2010; 38(3):445-463 www.ingentaconnect.com/content/tpp/pap/2010/00000038/00000003/art00008

33. Backman C, Zoutman DE. An integrative review of the current evidence on the relationship between hand hygiene interventions and the incidence of health care-associated infections. Am J Infection Control 2008; 36(5):333-348 www.ajicjournal.org/article/S0196-6553(07)00812-7/abstract

34. Trillis F, Eckstein EC. Contamination of hospital curtains with healthcare associated pathogens. Infect Cont Hosp Ep 2008; 29(11) www.jstor.org/stable/10.1086/591863

35. Clements A, Halton K. Overcrowding and understaffing in modern health-care systems: key determinants in methicillin-resistance Staphylococcus aureus transmission. Lancet Infect Dis 2008; 8(7):427-434 www.ncbi.nlm.nih.gov/pubmed/18582835

36. Cunningham JB, Kernoham WG. Bed occupancy and turnover interval as determinant factors in MRSA infections in acute settings in Northern Ireland: 1 April 2001 to 31 March 2003. J Hosp Infect 2005; 61(3):189-193 www.ncbi.nlm.nih.gov/pubmed/16153745

37. Dancer SJ, White LF. Measuring the effect of enhanced cleaning in a UK hospital: a prospective cross-over study. BMC Medicine 2009; 7:28 www.biomedcentral.com/1741-7015/7/28

38. Health Protection Agency, MRSA, Frequently Asked Questions www.hpa.org.uk/Topics/InfectiousDiseases/InfectionsAZ/StaphylococcusAureus/GeneralInformation/staphFrequentlyAskedQuestions/

39. Renal Patient View. https://www.renalpatientview.org/

Chapter 16 The unseen benefits of professional healthcare

1. De Craen AJM, Roos PJ. Effect of colour of drugs: systematic review of perceived effect of drugs and of their effectiveness. BMJ 1996; 313:1624 www.bmj.com/content/313/7072/1624.full

2. Blackwell B, Bloomfield S. Demonstration to medical students of placebo responses and non-drug factors. Lancet 1972; 229(7763):1279-1282 www.thelancet.com/journals/lancet/article/PIIS0140-6736(72)90996-8/abstract

3. Moseley JB, O'Malley K. A controlled trial of arthroscopic surgery for osteoarthritis of the knee. N Engl J Med 2002; 347:81-88 www.nejm.org/doi/full/10.1056/NEJMoa013259

4. Dimond EG, Kittle CF. Comparison of internal mammary artery ligation and sham operation for angina pectoris. Original Research Article Am J Cardiol 1960; 5(4):483-

486 www.ajconline.org/article/0002-9149(60)90105-3/abstract

5. Branthwaite A, Cooper P. Analgesic effects of branding in treatment of headaches. *BMJ* 1981; 282:1576-1578 www.ncbi.nlm.nih.gov/pmc/articles/PMC1505530/

6. Desharnais R, Jobin J. Aerobic exercise and the placebo effect: a controlled study. *Psychosomatic Medicine* 1993; 55(2): 149-154 www.psychosomaticmedicine.org/content/55/2/149.full.pdf

7. Stovner LJ, Oftedal G. Nocebo as headache trigger: evidence from a sham-controlled provocation study with RF fields. *Acta Neurologica* 2008; 117(s118): 67-71 onlinelibrary.wiley.com/doi/10.1111/j.1600-0404.2008.01035.x/abstract

8. Ivan Pavlov - Biography. Nobelprize.org. 28 Oct 2011 www.nobelprize.org/nobel_prizes/medicine/laureates/1904/pavlov-bio.html

9. Phillips DP, Ruth TE. Psychology and survival. *Lancet* 1993; 342(8880): 1142-1145 www.sciencedirect.com/science/article/pii/014067369392124C

10. Philips DP, Liu GC. The hound of the baskervilles effect: natural experiment on the influence of psychological stress on timing of death. *BMJ* 2001; 323(7327): 1443-1446 www.bmj.com/content/323/7327/1443.full

11. Ladwig KH, Roll G. Post-infarction depression and incomplete recovery 6 months after acute myocardial infarction. *Lancet* 1994; 343(8888):20-23 www.thelancet.com/journals/lancet/article/PIIS0140-6736(94)90877-X/abstract

12. Blumenthal J, Lett HS. Depression as a risk factor for mortality after coronary artery bypass surgery. *Lancet* 2003; 362(9384): 604-609 www.thelancet.com/journals/lancet/article/PIIS0140-6736(03)14190-6/fulltext

13. Lindstone SC, Schulzer M. Effects of expectation on placebo-induced dopamine release in Parkinson Disease. *Arch Gen Psychiatry* 2010; 67(8):857-865 archpsyc.ama-assn.org/cgi/content/full/67/8/857

14. Pollo A, Amanzio M. Response expectancies in placebo analgesia and their clinical relevance. *Pain* 2001; 93(1):77-84 www.painjournalonline.com/article/S0304-3959(01)00296-2/abstract

15. Grevert P, Albert LH. Partial antagonism of placebo analgesia by naloxone. Pain 1983; 16(2):129-143 www.sciencedirect.com/science/article/pii/0304395983902038

16. Hróbjartsson A, Gøtzsche PC. Placebo interventions for all clinical conditions. *Cochrane Db of Syst Rev* 2010, Issue 1. Art. No.: CD003974. onlinelibrary.wiley.com/doi/10.1002/14651858.CD003974.pub3/pdf/standard

17. Finniss DG, Kaptchuk TJ. Placebo effects: biological, clinical and ethical advances. *Lancet* 2010; 375(9715): 686-695 www.ncbi.nlm.nih.gov/pmc/articles/PMC2832199/

18. Kaptchuk TJ. Powerful placebo: the dark side of the randomised controlled trial. *Lancet* 1998; 351: 1722-1725 www.thelancet.com/journals/lancet/article/PIIS0140-6736(97)10111-8/fulltext

19. The Humble Humbug. *Lancet* 1954; 264(6833):321 www.sciencedirect.com/science/article/pii/S0140673654902457

20. Kaptchuk T, Kelley JM. Components of placebo effect: randomised controlled trial in patients with irritable bowel syndrome. *BMJ* 2008; 336:999 www.bmj.com/content/336/7651/999.full

21. Thomas KB. General practice consultations: is there any point in being positive? *BMJ* 1987; 294: 1200-1202 www.ncbi.nlm.nih.gov/pmc/articles/PMC1246362/?tool=pubmed

22. Little P, Everitt H. Observational study of effect of patient centeredness and positive approach on outcomes of general practice consultations. *BMJ* 2001; 323:908 www.bmj.com/content/323/7318/908.abstract

23. Hughes D. Consultation length and outcome in two group general practices. *J R Coll Gen Pract.* 1983 33(248): 143-144, 146-147 www.ncbi.nlm.nih.gov/pmc/articles/PMC1972718/

24. Campbell SM, Hann M. Identifying predictors of high quality care in English general practice: observational study. *BMJ* 2001 323:784 www.bmj.com/content/323/7316/784.full

25. Wilson A, Childs S. The relationship between consultation length, process and outcomes in general practice: a systematic review *Br Gen Pract.* 2002; 52(485):1012-1020 www.ncbi.nlm.nih.gov/pmc/articles/PMC1314474/?tool=pubmed

26. Stirling AM, Wilson P. Deprivation, psychological distress, and consultation length in general practice. *Br J Gen Pract.* 2001; 51(467)456-460 www.ncbi.nlm.nih.gov/pmc/articles/PMC1314026/

27. Mercer SW, Fitzpatrick B. More time for complex consultations in a high-deprivation practice is associated with increased patient enablement. *Br J Gen Pract.* 2007; 57(545): 960-966 www.ncbi.nlm.nih.gov/pmc/articles/PMC2084135/?tool=pubmed

28. Linde K, Ramirex G. St John's Wort for depression - an overview and meta-analysis of randomised clinical trials. *BMJ* 1996; 313:253 www.bmj.com/content/313/7052/253.full

29. Gratus C, Damery S. The use of herbal medicines by people with cancer in the UK: a systematic review of the literature. *QJM.* 2009; 102(12): 831-842 qjmed.oxfordjournals.org/content/102/12/831.abstract

30. Astin JA. Why patients use alternative medicine. *JAMA* 1998; 279(19): 1548-1553 jama.ama-assn.org/content/279/19/1548.full

31. Turner D, Tarrant C. Do patients value continuity of care in general practice? An investigation using stated preference discrete choice experiments. *J Health Serv Res Policy* 2007; 12(3):132-137 jhsrp.rsmjournals.com/content/12/3/132.long

32. Kearley KE, Freeman GK. An exploration of the value of the personal doctor-patient relationship in general practice. *Br Gen Pract.* 2001; 51(470): 712-718 www.ncbi.nlm.nih.gov/pmc/articles/PMC1314098/

33. Gill JM, Mainous AG. The role of provider continuity in preventing hospitalizations. *Arch Fam Med* 1998; 7:352-357 archfami.ama-assn.org/cgi/content/full/7/4/352

34. Cree M, Bell NR. Increased continuity of care associated with decreased hospital care and emergency department visits for patients with asthma. *Dis Manag* 2006; 9(1):63-71 www.ncbi.nlm.nih.gov/pubmed/16466343

35. Knight JC, Dowden JJ. Does higher continuity of family physician care reduce hospitalizations in elderly people with diabetes. *Popul Health Manag* 2009; 12(2):81-6 www.ncbi.nlm.nih.gov/pubmed/19361251

36. Burge F, Lawson B. Family physician continuity of care and emergency department use in end-of-life cancer care. Med Care 2003; 41(8):992-1001 www.ncbi.nlm.nih.gov/pubmed/12886178

37. Raddish M, Horn SD. Continuity of care: is it cost effective? *Am J Manag C* 1995; 5(6):727-734 www.ncbi.nlm.nih.gov/pubmed/10538452

38. Bamji AN. Southeast London – the unspoken problem. *BMJ* 2011; 342:d1765 www.bmj.com/content/342/bmj.d1765?tab=full

39. Mitchell AJ, Vaze A. Clinical diagnosis of depression in primary care: a meta-analysis. *Lancet* 2009; 374(9690):609-619 www.thelancet.com/journals/lancet/article/PIIS0140-6736(09)60879-5/abstract

40. Kai J, Crossland A. People with enduring mental health problems described the importance of communication, continuity of care, and stigma. *Evid Based Nurs* 2002;

5:93 ebn.bmj.com/content/5/3/93.full.pdf

41. McQueen D, St John Smith P. Psychiatric professionalism, multidisciplinary teams and clinical practice. *European Psychiatric Review*, 2009;2(2):50-56 www.touchpsychiatry. com/articles/psychiatric-professionalism-multidisciplinary-teams-and-clinical-practice

42. Craddock N, Antebi D. Wake-up call for British psychiatry. *Brit J Psychiat* 2008; 193:6-9 bjp.rcpsych.org/content/193/1/6.full

43. Simmons P, Hawley CJ. Service user, patient, client, user or survivor: describing recipients of mental health services. *The Psychiatrist Online* 2010; 34:20-23 pb.rcpsych. org/content/34/1/20

44. Propper C, Burgess S. Competition and quality: evidence from the NHS internal market. www.niesr.ac.uk/event/propper.pdf

45. Samuel M. NHS Market reforms pose risk to service, warn professionals. Communitycare.co.uk, 24th January 2011 www.communitycare.co.uk/ Articles/24/01/2011/116160/NHS-market-reforms-pose-risk-to-services-warn-

46. Health and social care bill 2011. Royal College of Psychiatrists, Second reading Briefing House of Commons. www.rcpsych.ac.uk/pdf/RCPsych%20Health%20 and%20Social%20Care%20Bill%20HOC%202nd%20Reading%20briefing%20-%20 final.pdf

Chapter 17 Getting back to the right kind of care

1. Williams B, Poulter NR. British Hypertension Society guidelines. *J Hum Hypertens* 2004; 18:139-185 www.bhsoc.org/pdfs/BHS_IV_Guidelines.pdf

2. McInnes GT. Drug treatment of prehypertension: Not now, not ever? Blood Pressure 2009; 18(6):304-307 informahealthcare.com/doi/abs/10.3109/08037050903416436

3. Pre-diabetes 'timebomb' warning. *BBC News*, October 2009 news.bbc.co.uk/1/hi/ health/8310297.stm

4. The United States of Diabetes: New Report Shows Half the Country Could Have Diabetes or Prediabetes at a Cost of $3.35 Trillion by 2020. United Health Group Newsroom. www.unitedhealthgroup.com/newsroom/news.aspx?id=36df663f-f24d-443f-9250-9dfdc97cedc5

5. Norris SL, Kansagara D. Screening adults for type 2 diabetes: a review of the evidence for the US preventive services Task Force. *Ann Intern Med* 2008; 148(11):855-68 www. annals.org/content/148/11/855.abstract

6. Lily M, Godwin M. Treating prediabetes with metformin. *Can Fam Physician* 2009; 55(4): 363-369 www.cfp.ca/content/55/4/363.full

7. Lowther M, Mordue A. Primary prevention of cardiovascular disease in Scotland: we must go further. The Heart Health Network Executive group. January 2006 www. vhscotland.org.uk/library/misc/NHS-CVD%20Full%20Doc.pdf

8. Marmot M. Social determinants of health inequalities. *Lancet* 365; 9464:1099-1104, 2005. www.thelancet.com/journals/lancet/article/PIIS0140-6736(05)71146-6/abstract

9. Fischer PM, Guinan KH. Impact of public cholesterol screening program. *Arch Intern Med* 1990; 150(12):2567-2572 archinte.ama-assn.org/cgi/content/abstract/150/12/2567

10. Croyle RT, Loftus EF. How well do people recall risk factor test results? Accuracy and bias among cholesterol screening participants. *Health Psychol* 2006; 25(3):425-32

11. NHS Health Scotland's 'Writing About Health Issues: Voices from Communities' (2004)

12. Ovarian Cancer: the recognition and initial management of ovarian cancer. NICE, Full Guideline, April 2011. www.nice.org.uk/cg122

13. Schorge JO. Modesitt SC. SGO white paper on ovarian cancer: Etiology, screening and surveillance. *Gynecologic Oncology* 2010; 119(1):7-17 www.sciencedirect.com/science/article/pii/S0090825810004300

14. Mai PL, Wentzensen N. Challenges related to developing serum-based biomarkers for early ovarian cancer detection. *Cancer Prev Res* 2011; 4:303 cancerpreventionresearch.aacrjournals.org/content/4/3/303.short

15. National Cancer Institute. Milestone (1971): National Cancer Act of 1971. dtp.nci.nih.gov/timeline/noflash/milestones/m4_nixon.htm

16. Temel J, Greer J. Early Palliative Care for Patients with Metastatic Non-Small-Cell Lung Cancer. *NEJM*, 2010, 363: 733-742 www.nejm.org/doi/pdf/10.1056/NEJMoa1000678

17. Hitchens C. Topic of Cancer. *Vanity Fair*, September 2011 www.vanityfair.com/culture/features/2010/09/hitchens-201009

18. Penson RT, Schapira L. Cancer as Metaphor. *The Oncologist* 2004; 9(6):708-716 theoncologist.alphamedpress.org/content/9/6/708.full

19. Petticrew M, Bell R. Influence of psychological coping on survival and recurrence in people with cancer: systematic review. *BMJ* 2002; 325:1066 www.bmj.com/content/325/7372/1066.1?view=long&pmid=12424165

20. Rapid Response to Petticrew M, Bell R. Influence of psychological coping on survival and recurrence in people with cancer: systematic review, *BMJ* 2002;325:1066.1 by Benjamin, HH 16/12/02

21. Temel JS, Greer JA. Early palliative care for patients with metastatic non-small-cell lung cancer. *N Engl J Med* 2010; 363:733-742

22. Comptroller and Auditor General. The provision of out-of-hours care in England, HC 2006; 1041

23. GP Daniel Ubani struck off over fatal overdose. *BBC News* June 2010 www.bbc.co.uk/news/10349596

24. Select Committee on Health Written Evidence. Memorandum by KernowDoc (GP13). www.publications.parliament.uk/pa/cm200304/cmselect/cmhealth/697/697we12.htm

25. Concerns over private GP Service. *BBC News* 21st September 2006 news.bbc.co.uk/1/hi/england/cornwall/5366262.stm

26. Overseas GP ordered to re-train. *BBC News* 30th October 2006 news.bbc.co.uk/1/hi/england/cornwall/6099494.stm

27. NHS 24 'changes' followed deaths. *BBC News* 30th January 2006 news.bbc.co.uk/1/hi/scotland/4663368.stm

28. Helpline advice 'linked to diabetic's death. *BBC News* 17th October 2001 news.bbc.co.uk/1/hi/england/1605250.stm

29. Travis A. Ministers face calls for apology as extent of 1970s 'virginity tests' revealed. *Guardian* 8th May 2011 www.guardian.co.uk/uk/2011/may/08/home-office-virginity-tests-1970s

30. The doctor cannot always tell: medical examination of the "intact" hymen. *Lancet* 1978: Feb 18i; 1(8060): 375–6. www.ncbi.nlm.nih.gov/pubmed/75407

31. McCartney M. Well enough to work? *BMJ* 2011; 342:d599 www.bmj.com/content/342/bmj.d599?tab=full

32. Faculty of Occupational Medicine. Good occupational medical practice. August 2010 www.facoccmed.ac.uk/library/docs/p_gomp2010.pdf

33. Harrington M. *An independent review of the work capability*. The Stationary Office. November 2010 www.dwp.gov.uk/docs/wca-review-2010.pdf

34. General Medical Council, Fitness to Practice Decisions. 4/10/10 www.gmc-uk.org/

concerns/hearings_and_decisions/fitness_to_practise_decisions.asp
35. Management Consultancies Association. Explores the myths about management consulting and the NHS. MCA News www.mca.org.uk/news/mca-explodes-myths-about-management-consulting-and-nhs
36. McKinsey & Co. Achieving world class productivity in the NHS 2009/10 –m 2013/14: Detailing the size of the opportunity. *Department of Health*, March 2009 www.dh.gov.uk/prod_consum_dh/groups/dh_digitalassets/documents/digitalasset/dh_116521.pdf?utm_source=Sign-Up.to&utm_medium=email&utm_campaign=201250-NHS+Institute+Alert+-+July+2010
37. Johnson S, Nolan F. Randomised controlled trial of acute mental health care by a crisis resolution team: the north Islington crisis study. *BMJ* 2005; 331(7517):599 www.bmj.com/content/331/7517/599.abstract
38. Johnson S, Nolan F. Randomised controlled trial of acute mental health care by a crisis resolution team: the north Islington crisis study. *BMJ* 2005, Rapid responses.
39. Gallegos NC, Dawson J. Risk of strangulation in groin hernias. *Br J Surg* 1991; 78(10):1171-3 www.ncbi.nlm.nih.gov/pubmed/1958976

Index

Index entries in **bold** are also to be found in the glossary on pages 295–298

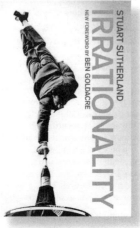
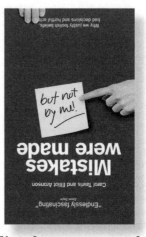
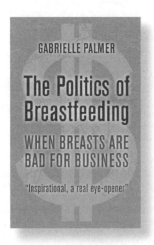
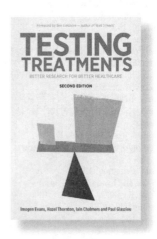